Research Skills for Nurses and Midwives

Sue Dyson and Peter Norrie

QUAY
BOOKS

A division of MA Healthcare Ltd

Quay Books Division, MA Healthcare Ltd, St Jude's Church, Dulwich Road, London
SE24 0PB

British Library Cataloguing-in-Publication Data
A catalogue record is available for this book

© MA Healthcare Limited 2013

ISBN-10: 1 85642 503 7
ISBN-13: 978 1 85642 503 2

Printed by Mimeo, Huntingdon, Cambridgeshire

Contents

Preface

When we wrote our first book, *Fundamental Aspects of Research for Nurses* (2010), we drew attention to the Prime Minister's Commission on The Future of Nursing and Midwifery in England, published on 2 March 2010, which stated that nurses and midwives must renew their pledge to society to deliver high-quality, compassionate care, thus placing quality of care at the top of the healthcare agenda. We wrote our book for student nurses who were committed to taking the first steps in research awareness in light of both this report and the changes taking place within nurse education, namely the move to an all-graduate profession. From September 2012 all pre-registration nursing programmes will have a degree-level target, requiring students to understand, use and undertake research as a prerequisite for thinking innovatively to influence system design in healthcare, and to impact positively on service delivery. Of course, midwifery has been ahead of nursing in this respect, having made a similar move in 2010, so we are delighted to have broadened the scope of this book to embrace both nurses and midwives in a joint research enterprise!

In the intervening two years, and with the change of government to a coalition in May 2010, the NHS has undergone some of the most radical restructuring in its history. The changes, completed in 2012, include the disassembling of the Strategic Health Authorities, the abolition of Primary Care Trusts, and the move by all NHS trusts to Foundation Trust status, with the commissioning of healthcare services becoming the responsibility of GPs working within Clinical Commissioning Groups (CCGs), overseen by the NHS Commissioning Board.

With regard to education and training, a function previously the responsibility of the SHAs, the Government within its White Paper 'Liberating the NHS: Developing the Healthcare Workforce' (DH, 2010a) proposed the establishment of Local Education and Training Boards (LETBs) to provide a forum for workforce development to support research and innovation, coordinate workforce planning activity, and commission education and training locally. A new body, Health Education England (HEE), has been commissioned to authorise and to support LETBs to promote high-quality education and training.

The overarching principles enshrined in the new legislation refer to the need to make the NHS more responsive, efficient and accountable, with a culture of research that is embedded at every level in both the NHS and in public health. The Health and Social Care Act 2012 places new duties on the Secretary of State for Health, the board and clinical commissioning groups to have regard to the need to promote research within the health service by explicitly providing the legal basis for research in the new NHS architecture. Under this provision the Secretary of State has a duty to promote research on matters relevant to the health service and the use in the health service of evidence obtained from research. Clearly, healthcare professionals, including nurses and midwives, who are at the forefront of healthcare delivery, need to be aware of and skilled in research in order to fulfil the requirements of the Health and Social Care Act, and in meeting the needs of patients and clients within the new landscape of health and social care.

This book aims to provide nurses and midwives with a sound theoretical knowledge base for understanding, critically appraising and undertaking research in all areas of health service provision. A comprehensive insight is provided into the philosophies, methodologies and methods used in social science research, where we locate the disciplines of nursing and midwifery, using examples from these distinct professions where appropriate. We include a new chapter which takes a pragmatic approach to research and offers a 'how to do' section, which nurses and midwives, beginning to engage with research for the first time, should find useful.

Once again we take the view that nurses and midwives are autonomous and curious learners, prepared to supplement their reading with other sources. To this end we offer suggestions throughout for further reading, plus a number of exercises to develop research skills. The book introduces student nurses and midwives to research, taking, as in our first edition, a conventional approach. Qualitative and quantitative methodologies are considered separately.

We begin in Chapter 1 with an overview of research philosophies and paradigms, including a consideration of mixed methods as a paradigm in and of itself, as opposed to simply a combination of methods. However, we recognise the place of mixed methods in our discussion of research design, strategy and data collection; therefore we refer to mixed methods throughout the book. We consider the importance of the research question and the literature review in determining the research design, before introducing quantitative, qualitative and mixed methodologies.

Chapter 2 provides an overview of qualitative research methods, focusing on ethnography, phenomenology, grounded theory, action research, feminist research and narrative methods. We illustrate the text with examples from published nursing and midwifery research where different research approaches have been used. Chapter 3 discusses methods for collecting qualitative data, including sampling strategies and methods for data analysis. Chapter 4 concludes the section on qualitative research, considering issues of quality and ethics in qualitative research.

Chapters 5 and 6 are concerned with quantitative research, including an exploration of the two most popular types: the classic scientific experiment and the use of surveys to explore populations. Quantitative data analysis is discussed in Chapter 7, which includes some exercises for those who are wary of statistics. In Chapter 8, we pay particular attention to mixed methods in research, in acknowledgment of the shift away from strict adherence to one particular approach to one which places the research question central in determining the most appropriate research design. The role of research as a source for evidence which can be used to develop healthcare is also addressed.

In Chapter 9 we take a 'how to do it' approach to preparing to write a research bid, writing a research proposal, and running a small-scale research project. We are of the belief that even though all nursing and midwifery courses cover research within the curriculum, often a theoretical approach is employed to the detriment of practical engagement in research. While it may not be feasible for undergraduate students to undertake empirical research for reasons of limited time and preclusive ethical issues, the consequences are that students may be well versed in the theory of research, but less so in how to carry it out. Dissertations are often library-based knowledge reviews, which compounds the problem. In essence, what we have is a perpetuation of the theory–practice gap. In Chapter 9 we show you, step by step, how to undertake a small research project from the initial stages of thinking about your project and looking for sources of funding, through to preparing and submitting your bid, thinking about good research governance, leading your research team, and finally sharing, through dissemination, your research findings.

We acknowledge our narrative is a theoretical account as, after all, we have written a research 'textbook'. Therefore we are reliant on you, the student, to put our ideas into practice, in other words to bridge the theory–practice gap and 'have a go' at doing research. Good luck!

SD and PN 2013

Acknowledgements

Sue would once again like to thank Simon Dyson for encouraging and supporting her efforts in all things work and life. Thanks to Emma and Matt McCartney and to Rehana Dyson, simply for being in my life.

Thank you to all the nursing students who, over the years, have been recipients of my research teaching. I hope to have made a difference, at least in terms of encouraging an interest in research.

Thanks to my mum who has in recent months helped me understand the meaning of dignity and fortitude – well done Mum. This book is dedicated to you.

Peter would like to thank his wife, Sarah and their children, Catherine and John, who are working their way through their A levels at the time of writing this second edition.

This is an expanded edition, so I will similarly expand the acknowledgments (apologies). My father Tom remains in our thoughts, but this is also a good opportunity to thank my stepmother Olive for her grammatical rectitude and kindness. Thanks again to my brother Alan, to my sister in-law Gwen, and to Roger and Sue Blackwell for enlivening our holidays and being unflagging advocates for their grandchildren.

Time has flown, but despite all (and possibly against my better judgment), I remain grateful to the late Carlos Castaneda, who introduced me to the *curandero*, Don Juan of New Mexico.

CHAPTER I

Understanding the language of research

Introduction

The preface to this book indicates the level of importance we place on an understanding of research for nurses and midwives. More now than ever, in the changing face of healthcare provision and delivery, it is imperative that nurses and midwives – indeed all those at the interface between service provision and service delivery – need to have a sound knowledge of research, including how to seek out and understand the best available evidence to underpin and facilitate the highest quality practice. Students of nursing and midwifery are keen to know their discipline, to become expert in that discipline and to make a difference to the patients, clients and families they come into contact with. In essence our students want to learn the 'tools of their trade', so to speak.

However, while we believe research to be the key to advancing knowledge of our subject, essential in helping make the right decisions regarding care delivery, and most important of all, vital to the creation of new knowledge within our discipline, our experience over many years of teaching research to nurses and midwives tells us that often the language of research is off-putting at the outset. When we introduce the topic of research early in the nursing and midwifery curriculum, students are not always ready to embrace it as an essential element of their discipline, being keen to learn the theory of their subject and to develop the necessary skills required for practice. What we have then, is a tension within the curriculum around when to introduce the topic of research, and how to teach it in a meaningful way.

The Nursing and Midwifery Council (NMC) requires students first and foremost to be competent and safe practitioners. An essential element of competency in practice is an understanding of the evidence base for practice at a level which ensures sound decision-making in relation to care delivery. This requires students to be able to read research, critically appraise what they are reading, and be confident that the methods described are the correct ones in relation to a given research problem or question; that the research process was carried out systematically, with due diligence paid to ethical issues, and that the findings can be relied upon as grounded in good research practice. These are our goals when teaching research within the nursing and midwifery curriculum; hence our book is based on achievement of these goals and written in such a way as to support research teaching, however and wherever it is manifest in your degree programme. While we accept that the language of research may be unfamiliar, we ask for your perseverance. You will become conversant with the language of research through reading this and other books about research for nurses and midwives.

As a nursing or midwifery student, you will be familiar with the language of nursing and midwifery practice, including well-known acronyms – for example BP (Blood Pressure), TPR (Temperature, Pulse and Respiration), CPR (Cardiopulmonary Resuscitation), A/N (Antenatal), Cx (Cervix) and CTG (Cardiotocograph). You may recall being introduced to this language early in your studies and wondering how you would ever come to understand and use it in a familiar and confident manner. Now that you are some way through your course, you will be familiar with this 'language of practice' and will have more than likely forgotten how it felt to be excluded and isolated by healthcare professionals who are experienced at using the language of practice as they go about their business. Moreover, like many healthcare professionals, you may view the acquisition of this language as a 'rite of passage' which students, yourself included, must traverse as part of the process of socialisation into the profession. We do not subscribe to this view, being of the mind that inaccessible language creates barriers that are both unnecessary and damaging to healthcare practice (including research), and in particular to nursing and midwifery students who are attempting to understand and undertake research perhaps for the first time. We will therefore take the time to describe as clearly as possible what we mean by certain terms and how we are using them, in order that you can begin to understand the language of research and its centrality to your practice.

In this chapter, we introduce the 'language of research', including research philosophies, research paradigms, methodologies and methods.

Research philosophies

Researchers are often asked to explain the philosophical basis for their research, whether this be funded research or research undertaken as part of research degree studies. Philosophy is generally concerned with questions about reality, existence, values, reason, mind and language; whereas research philosophy is concerned with how the world is perceived and how best we can come to understand the world. By this we mean to what extent researchers believe that, on the one hand, we are active in creating or shaping the social world in which we live, or on the other hand, that the social world exists independently of what we may think of it. On first reading this paragraph you might already feel lost, thinking that research is too deep, complicated and complex, and not for you. This is understandable if you are new to research and has much to do with unfamiliar terminology for what are actually quite straightforward ways of thinking about important questions and how best to find the answers. While research may be detailed, can be complex, and may involve groups of people with very different views about a particular issue, it is nevertheless something you can undertake. The most important point to make here is that you can come to understand the philosophical basis of research and begin to understand how your own worldview shapes the kinds of research you may want to undertake.

It is important to note that the approach advocated in this chapter is not without its critics. Authors have pointed out that holding fast to a philosophical position at the outset can inhibit our understanding, as it precludes the possibility of an alternative viewpoint (Dyson and Brown, 2006). For example, if we were to ask student nurses and midwives for their views on being supported in the practice setting by academic teachers we would be taking the philosophical position that it is possible to understand the social world in which the student lives, and therefore we would be prepared to accept the student's view on this matter. The alternative position is that it is not possible to understand how the student perceives the world with any degree of certainty; therefore we need other forms of knowledge to answer the question posed in order that we can be sure of or convinced by the information (data) gathered. Our method of enquiry, should we view the world this way, might be to collect information (data) about how many times students were visited in practice by academic teachers, how long these encounters lasted, and whether or not a formal assessment was conducted.

In spite of criticisms of an approach where the researcher has a predetermined idea of how we can come to know the world, an advantage is that the researcher can more readily apply a structured and logical approach to designing and carrying out the research. Certainly, for beginning researchers this is a most useful approach. However, it is important (and indeed the position taken in this book) that the beginning researcher strives to keep an open mind. Dyson and Brown (2006) sum up this position when suggesting that researchers who adopt a philosophical viewpoint at the outset may use it as a cloak against other philosophical positions. While this approach has the attraction of consistency, it may lead the researcher to believe they have found the one '*true*' philosophical position, to the exclusion of all others (Dyson and Brown, 2006, p. 3).

When placed in the context of research, philosophy is about how we can come to know the social world in order to understand why practitioners and users of health and social care services think and subsequently act in the way they do. For example, we may ask the question why, in spite of evidence to the contrary, do individuals continue to engage in unhealthy practices such as smoking, excessive drinking and overeating? Similarly, why do a significant number of health and social care practitioners engage in similar practices when we could argue that although the first group may be excused through lack of exposure to health-promoting messages, the second group should really know better, through exposure to specific health education – some of which they may actually teach! Of course, this is to oversimplify what is occurring, as we know there are many factors influencing individual health behaviour. For researchers in health and social care, interested in exploring these phenomena or manifestations of behaviour, we need to know something about research philosophy if we are to understand the fundamental problems for practitioners and users of health and social care services and to ask the right questions in the right ways.

Until recently, it was generally accepted that there are two main ways of coming to know the social world, by which we mean the world inhabited by social beings or communities as opposed to the world of the individual. These distinct philosophies gave rise to two paradigms (patterns of thought) referred to as the positivist and interpretivist paradigms. However, researchers now recognise the place of mixed methods research (in particular the notion of pragmatism within mixed methods) as offering an alternative but legitimate paradigm within research (we will return to this later). Before we look at the characteristics of positivism, interpretivism and mixed methods, we need to consider exactly what we mean by a paradigm and how we have arrived at a position whereby researchers generally associate themselves, rightly or wrongly, with one or another paradigm. This is important, as we need to be able to articulate how our view has informed our subsequent decisions about research design to those who share our interests and are, in turn, interested in our research findings.

Research paradigms

A paradigm is a set of assumptions, concepts, values and practices constituting a view of reality. In terms of research a paradigm represents a view shared by a scientific community about how we can come to know the essence of things (*ontology*) and how we can come to know what is true, and what is false (*epistemology*). Over time, scientific communities have come to hold a common set of assumptions and values and to follow certain rules in pursuit of solutions to problems in the real world.

The EQUANS study

The writing that follows will draw on an example of research to provide some context to what might otherwise be a quite abstract discussion. Research undertaken for the National Sickle Cell and Thalassaemia Screening Programme (a scientific community) sought to establish whether the costly processes of antenatal screening of women for sickle cell and thalassaemia genes could be targeted by focusing on women who answered an ethnicity question and placed themselves into a group at higher risk of carrying such genes (economically but potentially inequitable), or whether all women, irrespective of an answer to an ethnicity question, should be offered such screening (equitable but economically expensive), comparing different population groups undergoing different treatments across different periods (Dyson *et al.*, 2006).

The assumption underpinning the first phase of the Ethnicity and Antenatal Screening Study (EQUANS) was that it would be possible to answer the research question by undertaking a randomised controlled trial (a positivistic paradigm: more of this later). In the EQUANS study a category-based ethnicity screening question was shown to be more effective than a binary plus open-ended question. Study data were analysed using statistical tests to understand whether an ethnicity question would be sufficiently valid and reliable as a screening question to ascertain risk status for sickle cell/thalassaemia in an antenatal screening programme.

The paradigm underpinning this research is positivism, because the researchers do not intend to ask the participants (in this phase of the EQUANS study) about their experiences, feelings or views regarding screening, but rather have chosen to gather numerical data, which can be subjected to statistical tests to measure the error rate between midwife and participant (pregnant women) assignment of ethnicity. In utilising an essentially positivistic approach the EQUANs study was able to show that using the more effective question, 5.74% (CI 2.34–11.46%) of significant haemoglobinopathies will be missed in a selective screening programme, and 4.33% (CI 2.63–6.68%) of replies to an ethnicity screening question will be unreliable when compared to information given upon re-interview (Dyson *et al.*, 2006).

Positivism

Positivists believe the goal of science is to uncover the truth. Consequently, a positivist would view science as a means of getting at the truth in order to understand the world well enough to predict and control it. Stereotypically, scientists are depicted wearing white coats and based in laboratories. This image was certainly true in the past, supported by popular imagery such as television and film. Positivistic scientists are interested in observing what can be seen (phenomena), describing what is seen and measuring what is seen. Knowledge of anything beyond the observed, described and measured is impossible to the positivist. Taking this a step further, a positivist would argue those things not directly observed (for example, thoughts, feelings and emotions) are not legitimate subjects for study. A fundamental positivist would argue what cannot be measured is irrelevant. Positivists believe empiricism (the pursuit of knowledge by observation and experiment) to be central to scientific endeavour. Hence positivistic research is usually of an experimental design and uses quantitative approaches to data collection such as those described in the first phase of the EQUANs study (Dyson *et al.*, 2006).

Post-positivism

In recent times (since the mid-20th century) thinking about science has undergone a marked shift, with a rejection of the positivistic view that science works through observation and experiment and that this is distinctly different from how everyday life is experienced. In an era now defined as post-positivism scientists do not view scientific reasoning and common sense reasoning as mutually exclusive, but as part of the same process, namely an attempt to make sense of the world.

Scientific research relies on results, which are verifiable, accurate and consistent. Although common sense reasoning does not always proceed in a systematic way, it is often underpinned by observation and measurement. When thinking about everyday healthcare practice you will be able to recall occasions when you knew your patient's condition had deteriorated long before any clinical observations confirmed your suspicions. This is intuitive practice, and while not underpinned by evidence in the scientific sense, it is based on observations of similar patients with similar conditions over considerable periods. Indeed, Patricia Benner's classic work recognised that nurses arrive at an understanding of patient care over time, not only through a sound educational base, but from a multitude of experiences (Benner, 1984).

The most common form of post-positivist thinking is a philosophy known as critical realism, which attempts to reconcile the position taken by the positivist and that taken by the interpretivist. By way of an example, the second phase of the EQUANS study sought to understand from the pregnant women and their midwives what it is like to be asked and to ask an ethnicity question, during the first meeting of mother and her midwife, namely at the 'booking in' antenatal visit. The research team observed the interaction between mother and midwife and followed this up with an interview. The midwife was asked to describe the experience of asking pregnant women to describe their ethnicity in order to assess their risk of carrying genes associated with sickle cell disorder, and the pregnant women were asked to describe their experience of being asked an ethnicity question. The assumption underpinning this phase of the EQUANS study was a belief in the possibility of knowing another person's experience by asking that person to describe their experiences, and furthermore that this is a legitimate form of knowledge.

Interpretivism

As we have shown, the positivist researcher places emphasis on explanation, prediction and control. Enquiry using a positivistic approach answers questions that readily lend themselves to numerical measurement: for example, how many nursing and midwifery students use the library facilities at the weekend, and during which hours. These types of questions are important, as we need to be able to predict library usage in the future and to ensure supply can meet demand.

Important questions around the provision of healthcare services lend themselves to positivistic enquiry: for example, the length of time that patients and clients may be waiting for healthcare services. Answers to these questions are important in order to ensure that users of services receive the care they need in a timely fashion in the most cost-effective manner (you can think of many more important questions that lend themselves to this type if enquiry). What positivist approaches to enquiry cannot tell us is how the individual, whether student or service user (or indeed individuals in any social situation) perceives, interprets and makes sense of the situation.

To continue with the earlier examples, we might also want to know what students think about the library's weekend opening times, how this relates to their view of the university as a whole, and how it helps or hinders their overall study experience. Similarly, we need to know how service users feel about waiting for healthcare services, how this influences their experience of health (for example pregnant women experiencing antenatal care) and illness (for example patients experiencing coronary heart disease), and how they make sense of these experiences now and the likely impact of this on future health behaviour. Collecting numerical data to help predict and control will not shed light on these important questions. For this we need a different approach, namely an interpretive approach to enquiry.

The interpretive approach to enquiry links with philosophy and the human sciences. Researchers adopting an interpretivist approach think of individuals as existing not in isolation, but as inseparable from the wider context of their everyday lives. Students at university are not separate from the wider social context in which they live; they bring the context of their lives with them, and their experience of university occurs within this context. Each student will have a unique university experience, while at the same time sharing similar experiences with other students. Similarly, service users and patients bring the wider context of their lives with them to the healthcare setting, and this shapes and colours their experience of health and illness.

Social scientists are concerned for the most part with understanding the unique world in which the individual lives. While social scientists may use numerical data to inform their enquiry, emphasis is placed on understanding the world of the 'other' rather than explaining that world. Social scientists use interpretivist approaches to gain access to an individual's experience and perception of reality. Social scientists are interested in qualitative expression, rather than quantitative measurement. Consequently, interpretivist researchers use qualitative approaches to data collection.

Critical realism

Critical realism recognises that observation is always fallible and prone to error; therefore theory can always be revised. The critical realist is critical of our ability to know reality with any degree of certainty. Of importance to the critical realist is the idea of holding fast to an attempt to get it right about reality rather than uncovering the truth, simply because we may never know the truth for sure.

A critical realist will attempt to use multiple methods (triangulation) to observe and measure reality in an effort to understand what is happening in the real world. These varying methods may have different types of errors within them; you may have your view of the world based on your experience and I will have mine. For example, you may observe the practice of your colleagues as being different from what you understand as good practice based on what has been taught in the classroom setting. In essence, this is the theory–practice gap, so often alluded to. Practitioners often refer to this as the reality of practice. Our view is that in order to make sense of the reality of practice and to maintain the integrity or truthfulness required for good practice, one must first know with a degree of certainty the evidence for a particular practice, in order to 'hold fast' to your view of what constitutes best practice. While your perception will not change, you may come to understand the perspective of the other person, recognising it as constructed by their experience. Thus you will be well placed to influence not only your practice but the practice of others for the better.

Critical realism allows multiple fallible sources to get a better view of what is going on by acknowledging that all observations, including those of scientists, are theory-laden and biased by experience. At this point you may well be asking how we can conduct research in any objective way if we allow multiple sources to inform our understanding of what is occurring (the phenomenon being studied), especially since these have been shown to be very different. A critical realist would argue that objectivity is not exclusive to an individual but rather belongs to a social group. Objectivity is what we strive for when we criticise each other's work. In this sense, we may never achieve true objectivity, but as a community of truth seekers we can approach objectivity through scrutiny. Those theories that survive scrutiny are theories we can be most confident in.

For example, if we listen to our patients, who consistently tell us they fear going into hospital because of the risk of infection, we can develop a theory that patients are concerned about the risk of hospital-acquired infection. The actual risk may be low in terms of total number of patients admitted to hospital. However, anxiety and stress are known to lower resistance to disease, making it more likely that anxious patients will be less resistant to infection. Using multiple sources of evidence, some of which may be fallible, allows for theory to be generated. For example, patients whose fears and anxieties around hospital-acquired infection are recognised and addressed are less likely to succumb to infection in the hospital setting.

Mixed methods

You may recall that we mentioned a third philosophical position, which has gained in popularity since the 1980s because it bridges the divide between the positivist and interpretivist philosophical positions. Mixed methods research, also known as mixed methodology or multi-methodology, focuses on research questions that call for real-life contextual understandings, multi-level perspectives and cultural influences, whereby rigorous quantitative and qualitative research methods are integrated to draw on the strengths of each, thereby framing the investigation within the philosophical and theoretical positions of both approaches in the pursuit of pragmatism (linking theory and practice).

Mixed methods research has been seen as transformative in being able to use pragmatism to employ what works, using diverse approaches, giving primacy to the importance of the research problem and question. Critics of mixed methods are usually those who hold fast to a philosophical tradition, believing it impossible to hold more than one philosophical position as the 'true' position at the same time, thereby making the mixing of methods at best ineffective and at worst untenable.

In summary, we have looked at philosophies of research as a starting point for thinking about how we might undertake research to underpin our practice: an important part of the role and responsibilities of nurses and midwives to service users and patients, which is as important as updating clinical knowledge. We began by thinking about how we might come to know the social world in which we live. It is generally accepted that there are three philosophical positions, two of which have opposing views, namely positivism, with its emphasis on the observable and objective way of knowing the social world, and interpretivism, a subjective view of knowing the social world. We introduced the concept of critical realism, where emphasis is placed on understanding the 'real' world, as it is experienced by those we are interested in knowing more about.

A third philosophical position (often subscribed to by the critical realist) is said to underpin 'mixed methods', which attempts to bridge the divide between the two well-established philosophies in the name of pragmatism. Whichever view is subscribed to on a personal level, the key point is to think about the research question, i.e. what do we want to know, and to design the research study in a way that best enables the question to be answered.

For example, a researcher seeking to understand students' experience of using the library would design a study grounded in interpretivism, whereby it is possible to come to know what it is like to use the library from the students' perspective. On the other hand, a researcher wishing to know peak usage time for the library would design a study within the positivist paradigm and observe students using the library during certain times of the day. Both are useful pieces of research, but for different reasons and for different audiences. It is useful for library staff to know how students experience the library, so that they can facilitate improvements. However, if the question is one of how to make the best use of available resources, a different audience will be interested in the results, namely those responsible for resourcing the library and capital expenditure. A critical realist might use a mixed methods approach in order to understand the realities of library services for users within the context of an organisations diminishing resources. What is suitable for one research study may not be suitable for another depending on the question and the targeted audience for the research findings.

The research question

The research process begins when there is a problem in need of a solution, with the aim being to design a research study that will enable the problem to be solved. This is true irrespective of the preferred methodology, be it quantitative or qualitative. Identifying research problems in healthcare is relatively simple, as most of us have worked in the field in some capacity. Consequently, our exposure to and experience of healthcare situations means that we are best placed to identify problems of interest to the real world of healthcare practice.

Often the identification of a research problem arises from a disagreement or discussion: for example, how nursing and midwifery care should be organised, how health services should be delivered, or what treatments and care patients and clients require or desire. The researcher then translates these disagreements or discussions into a researchable question and proceeds to design a research study using the most appropriate methodology to address the research question. In general, research ideas and questions arise from existing theories or previous research. Similarly, research questions in nursing and midwifery can arise from everyday practice, past nursing and midwifery research, or theory.

One of the most fruitful areas for research ideas is everyday nursing and midwifery practice. Practitioners continually have to make decisions about how to organise care, when to alert medical staff to a change in a patient's condition, when there are issues for a mother in labour, and (more often these days) how to make best use of available resources. Practitioners will be constantly observing and reflecting on their practice and the practice of others and thinking about how best to solve clinical and practice problems. Situations and experiences such as these, and many others you can think of, can be turned into research questions with the aim of improving practice for the benefit of patients and clients.

Previous research studies are another source of research ideas and questions because they often recommended further research in a subject. An interesting feature of research is that it tends to generate more questions than it answers. In addition, from reviewing and analysing research articles as a student you may have found issues in the published research that are problematic. In this case, your critique may be a good starting place to propose further research, which in turn adds to the body of nursing and midwifery knowledge.

The necessity to test or build theory is another source of research ideas and/or questions. Theory is an explanation of how a phenomenon operates and why. Theory serves the purpose of making sense out of current knowledge by integrating and summarising what is currently known. Theory building goes beyond what is currently known and attempts to suggest new relationships and make new predictions. New research studies can confirm or disconfirm nursing and midwifery theory.

Identifying a research idea or problem does not mean that this will be the exact focus of your research study, because the issue may have already been researched sufficiently for theory to become accepted practice. Alternatively, you may have identified a broad topic area from experience or observations of everyday practice, from previous research or from existing theory that now requires a different or innovative approach to investigation. Identification of the research topic is the beginning of the sequential process that leads to the generation of the research question and culminates in the design of the research study. Refining the research question and designing the research study require a review of the research literature.

The literature review

Once the research topic has been identified, the next stage is to find out what is already known about the area to be investigated. The aim here is to refine the topic into a researchable question, to ensure that the research study will add to what is known about the issue, and to avoid repeating the limitations of previous research studies.

Reading and reviewing the literature to find out what is known about a subject can involve a number of sources, such as previous research studies published in academic journals, anecdotal accounts of practice, or textbooks and documentary sources. Reference can also be made to sources such as radio, television and audiovisual media, such as slides and photographs. Online databases are a good source of information, as are Internet sources. However, the researcher should exercise caution and maintain a degree of scepticism regarding the validity and reliability of online sources until the quality of the material can be verified. Cross-checking and referring to sources other than the Internet (for example published papers), is one way of doing this.

The literature review also serves the purpose of providing a rationale for a research study. Researchers may claim that the reason for undertaking research is that little or no research exists in a particular area. In this case, the literature review provides evidence that this is in fact the case, with literature cited that relates to the proposed study, but drawn from a broader subject area. The researchers are then able to justify the need for more focused research. A further reason for undertaking a literature review is to provide a context for the proposed research. In this case, the literature review locates the current study within the context of what is already known in the subject area.

The value of information to a given research study depends on whether it is a primary or secondary source. Original literature is a primary source: for example, a government report or textbook, or where the researcher has access to the original publication of a research study. Secondary sources are those where a person other than the person who undertook the original research reports on research. Both sources are useful. However, it is important where possible to draw on primary sources, as secondary sources may misinterpret, misreport or distort the original literature. Where it is not possible to acquire the primary source, secondary sources are useful in shedding light on or conveying the essence of the original source. The researcher must make it clear, using recognised referencing techniques, whether sources of material are primary or secondary, and should as far as possible avoid over-using secondary sources.

The extent of a literature review depends on the target audience. For example, the review might be undertaken as part of original research for a programme of study, such as a Master's degree or a PhD. In these circumstances, the extent of the literature review is constrained by convention. In externally funded research projects the extent of the literature review may be determined by available resources and the requirements of funding bodies. Researchers will not be able to write about all the literature concerning a subject and will need to make a judgement regarding what *must* be included, what *could* be included, and what can reasonably be *omitted*. In most cases there will be literature that is integral to the proposed research and is deemed a classic text, the omission of which would seriously affect the integrity of the review. In most literature reviews, the researchers refer to the scope of the review, indicating the period it covers, the countries covered and any other distinguishing features of the review.

We note here that some research studies consist entirely of a systematic review of the literature, whereby the researcher reviews and evaluates what is already published in a given area. Systematic reviews are an accepted research approach and can serve as research in their own right or as an integral part of the literature review for a new study.

Research methodologies

A research paradigm is a worldview including philosophical and socio-political issues, whereas a research methodology is a general approach to scientific inquiry involving preferences for broad components of the research process (Teddlie and Tashakkori, 2009). Research methodology refers to the principles guiding the researcher's choice of strategy and procedure for undertaking research. A researcher chooses a methodological approach to carrying out the research, based on a preferred research philosophy. As we have seen, research philosophy is a set of beliefs about how we can come to know the world, namely positivist or interpretivist. Positivistic methodologies are quantitative in nature, whereas interpretivist methodologies are qualitative in nature. Mixed methods, as the name implies, use a combination of quantitative and qualitative methodologies in order to address the research question in the most effective manner. Methodology then, is a general approach to a scientific inquiry.

Quantitative methodology

Quantitative methodology is used in research studies in which the data are analysed numerically. Relatively large data sets are used, which are representative of the broad population being studied. Statistical tools (which are often complex) are used to analyse the data in order to give additional meaning to the research findings. Statistical tests are used to describe data in a meaningful way or to infer from the study population the things that may pertain to the whole of that population.

Quantitative approaches to research are useful in understanding trends and are used in the field of public health to look at underlying patterns of disease and to predict future requirements for the provision of healthcare services. Quantitative research will not explain or shed light on how individuals think about healthcare services, or indeed what they prefer to be available. Without this information, healthcare planners may make inappropriate choices for service provision, to the detriment of patient satisfaction.

Qualitative methodology

Qualitative methodology is used in research which seeks to understand the individual's point of view. Large data sets are not necessary, as the aim is not to generalise or infer from the findings to the whole of the population for that study. Rather, the aim is to understand from the individual respondent how the phenomenon is experienced. The sample size may be relatively small in qualitative research, depending on the method of data collection. Data from qualitative research are not subject to statistical tests, as respondents usually tell of their experiences, or feelings, in their own words. Common methods for collecting qualitative data are interviews and focus groups, transcribed verbatim (word for word).

Conclusion

This chapter looked at research philosophy and research paradigms. We have learnt that researchers usually hold a philosophical position about how we can come to know the social world around us. On the one hand, the social world is understood only through knowledge from direct observation and measurement, while on the other hand the social world can be understood through knowledge from accounts of individual experience.

We considered the centrality of both the research question and the literature review in decisions about research design. Researchers who come from a scientific background usually, although by no means exclusively, are consistent with a set of assumptions, concepts, values, and practices consistent with the positivist paradigm. These researchers generally undertake research using quantitative methodologies, which involve collecting numerical data. In contrast, researchers coming from a social science background, including health and social care, will more than likely adhere to a set of assumptions, concepts, values and practices consistent with the interpretivist paradigm. These researchers generally undertake research using qualitative methodologies, which involve collecting descriptive data. We considered the concept of mixed methods, describing this approach as bridging the gap between the well-recognised philosophies of positivism and interpretivism, and often adopted by critical realists in an effort to understand or come to know reality. In the next chapter, we provide an overview of qualitative research methods.

Further reading

Dyson, S. and Brown, B. (2006) *Social Theory and Applied Health Research.* Open University Press, Berkshire.

Howell, K. E. (2013) *An Introduction to the Philosophy of Methodology.* Sage, London.

Lincoln, Y. and Guba, E. (1985) *Naturalistic Inquiry.* Sage, London.

Midgeley, M. (2001) *Science and Poetry.* Routledge, London.

Ridley, D. (2012) *The Literature Review: A Step-by-Step Guide for Students.* 2nd edn. Sage, London.

Sim, J. and Wright, C. (2000) *Research in Health Care. Concepts, Designs and Methods.* Nelson Thornes, Cheltenham.

CHAPTER 2

Qualitative research: an overview of methods

Introduction

Qualitative research encompasses a wide range of methodologies and methods. However, all qualitative work is interpretive in nature. A key aspect of qualitative research is a reliance on unstructured information to answer key questions. In this sense, qualitative research does not rely on statistics or numbers. Consequently, the methods used to gather data (information) are usually interviews (structured, semi-structured and unstructured), focus groups and analysis of documentary evidence, including diaries, video clips, oral histories and testimonials – indeed, any unstructured information.

Any method of data collection that seeks to answer the 'why' and not the 'how' of its subject is more than likely to be qualitative in nature. The key features of qualitative research are its focus on natural settings; its interest in meanings, perspectives and understandings; sharp emphasis on process; and a concern with inductive analysis and grounded theory. Qualitative research as a method of inquiry is used in many disciplines. However, qualitative methods lend themselves particularly well to the social sciences, where researchers are concerned with gathering an in-depth understanding of human behaviour and the reasons for that behaviour. Qualitative research is not just about what people think, but is concerned with why they think it. Qualitative methods are designed to 'draw out' research participants' opinions in order to better understand motivations and feelings underlying behaviour.

Examples of nursing and midwifery research using a variety of qualitative approaches are provided in boxes throughout this chapter with suggestions for

Box 2.1

Kennedy *et al.* (2006) were interested to know about the practice of midwifery from a diverse sample of midwives. These researchers were of the view that while the practice of midwifery reflects the spectrum of diversity among midwives and the women they serve, the actual composition of midwives in the American College of Nurses and Midwives (ACNM) does not reflect the diversity of the women for whom they provide care.

To answer the research question the investigators utilised small group interviews and videotape collection of data and were able to identify four major themes including the worldview of midwifery through the lens of diversity, the experience of diversity, the midwifery strategies rooted in diversity and the legacy for the profession of midwifery. The researchers came to the conclusion there must be purposeful action by every individual in the profession, as well as the collective voice of midwifery, to identify barriers to inclusiveness and to foster a culture of diversity through respect, recruitment and mentoring (Kennedy et al. (2006, p. 85). The approach to addressing the research question clearly lent itself to qualitative methodology in that the midwives needed to be given a 'voice' in order to share their perspectives and understandings within their 'natural setting', in this case, within their own practice.

further reading given at the end of the chapter. We begin with two examples which illustrate how researchers, first in the context of midwifery, and second in nursing, have utilised qualitative approaches to answer questions of interest to their respective clinical practice.

There are a number of approaches to conducting qualitative research. While these are all interpretivist in nature, the approaches taken to data collection and subsequent data analysis are different. We now consider the major approaches to qualitative research widely used in the social sciences, particularly in nursing and midwifery: ethnography, phenomenology, grounded theory, action research, feminist theory and narrative research. A summary of each approach is provided at the end of each account.

Box 2.2

Ashing-Giwa *et al.* (2002) investigated the breast cancer experiences of African American, Asian American, Latina and Caucasian breast cancer survivors. A total of 102 breast cancer survivors from different ethnic groups participated in focus groups exploring differences in types of treatment, quality of life and ongoing concerns after treatment.

Through invitation, the women talked about their experiences and the researchers were able to show that there are indeed differences in treatments offered to women from different ethnic groups. Women of colour are less likely to receive adjuvant therapies, including radiation and chemotherapy, and more likely to receive mastectomies. Furthermore, while all women experience similar concerns, (for example recurrence of the cancer and worry about family, body image and sexual health), women of colour reported their spiritual beliefs and practices to be central to their coping.

The results of this qualitative study, whereby the women were given a 'voice' and an opportunity to talk about individual experiences of breast cancer, provided invaluable information for healthcare providers and future survivors of breast cancer about the impact of culture on survivorship, in ways that a quantitative study would not.

Qualitative methods

Ethnography

A good place to begin to think about different approaches to qualitative research is to look first at ethnography, because it is considered the oldest of the qualitative approaches. The purpose of ethnography is to provide a detailed description of everyday life events or 'thick description', and for this reason much qualitative research is ethnographic in nature. Ethnography is the research method of anthropology and as such can trace its history back to the Greeks and Romans, who described their travels in detail (thick description). In its purest sense, ethnography is a description of the people or a writing of a culture (Holloway, 1997).

Ethnography is both research process and research outcome, in that the researcher conducts an ethnographic study, but also produces an interpretation of the culture under investigation. *Culture*, used here in its broadest sense, refers to a system of knowledge shared by a relatively large group of people. Ethnographers may study many different cultures, for example organisational culture, business culture, cultural practice in nursing, cultural practice in midwifery and culture in nurse education. What the ethnographer is concerned with, whatever the culture studied, is the web of meaning (Geertz, 1973) or the cultural constructions in which the members of that particular culture live. The ultimate aim of the ethnographer is to observe, record, analyse and then interpret the information collected (data), to gain the meaning of the culture itself with the ultimate goal of initiating dialogues between cultures.

Imagine an ethnographic study which aimed to describe in detail the cultural practices of nurses working in Accident and Emergency (A&E) departments and to make sense of those practices as understood by the nurses themselves. The ethnographic researcher, immersed in the world of A&E, is best placed to observe, analyse and interpret what it means to work under pressure, to meet the targets, and to ensure that patients do not remain in A&E longer than four hours from admission to transfer (DH, 2000). Ethnography, with its emphasis on the '*emic*' or insider's point of view is able to generate a cultural understanding of A&E practice, thus enabling critical categories and meanings to emerge rather than imposing these by using approaches that are essentially '*etic*' or from an outsider's perspective. Similarly, if a researcher wished to understand the cultural practices of midwives working in midwifery units, then an ethnographic study would serve this purpose.

Box 2.3

Hughes *et al.* (2002) wanted to improve understanding of local midwifery morale in order to inform the development and reorganisation of a maternity unit and to enhance midwifery involvement in strategic planning. The researchers adopted a critical ethnographic approach, which they describe as being focused on power and how this is distributed in a cultural setting. Focus groups were employed for data collection and the researchers, by emphasising an essentially 'emic' or insider point of view (in this case that of the midwives who were affected by working conditions in the midwifery unit in question), were able to identify that staffing levels, working relationships and organisational issues were particularly important areas affecting midwifery morale.

In summary, an ethnographic exploration is one developed through close exploration of a number of sources of data, usually collected over time, on which the researcher comes to rely to develop a cultural frame of reference. Ethnography has been successfully used in nursing and midwifery research, where the key questions relate to the study of culture, for example the study of institutions or a professional group, both of which are cultural phenomena.

Hammersley (1990) provides us with a useful summary of the features of ethnographic research are useful in helping us recognise ethnographic research:

■ People's behaviour is studied in everyday contexts, rather than under experimental conditions created by the researcher.
■ Data are gathered from a range of sources, but usually from observation and relatively informal conversations.
■ The approach to data collection is unstructured and does not normally follow a detailed plan set up at the beginning; nor are the categories used for interpreting what people say and do predetermined or fixed. This does not mean the research is unsystematic; rather that initial data are collected in as raw a form as possible, and on as wide a front as is feasible.
■ The focus is usually a single setting or group of relatively small scale.
■ Data analysis involves interpretation of the meanings and functions of human actions and mainly takes the form of verbal descriptions and expla-

nations, with quantifications and statistical analysis, if present, taking a subordinate role at best.

There are a number of options available to ethnographic researchers in terms of collecting data. However, what is required is a commitment to getting as close to the subject observed as possible. It is essential to collect data in their natural setting, and to report these data in a factual and descriptive manner. The points of view of the recipients are integral, and an absolute commitment to accurate and true reporting is essential to ethnographic research. Once the rules of good ethnographic research are observed, the researcher can design the study and subsequent methods for collecting data in a way that best serves the situation.

There are usually two approaches taken to data collection in ethnography, both of which involve observation. However, observation is either participant or non-participant, depending on the context in which the research is taking place, access to the participants, ethical issues and available resources. In addition, within the decision to choose either participant or non-participant observation, an ethnographic researcher will have to decide on the extent of the participation or non-participation: for example, the researcher may be immersed in a culture, or be an observer of a culture. Alternatively, the researcher may take a position that is somewhere between the two.

Phenomenology

In Chapter 1 we looked at the philosophical positions taken by researchers when attempting to think about the social world in which we live. We considered the scientific or positivist approach, which seeks to understand the world through recording as evidence only that which is directly observed, and discounting all that cannot be directly observed. In contrast to this view is phenomenology, which by its very nature is essentially relative and subjective. We now move on to consider phenomenology in detail and discuss why researchers might choose a phenomenological approach when undertaking qualitative research.

Phenomenology has overlaps with other approaches to qualitative research, in particular ethnography, which we have previously considered. However, phenomenology is unique in that the point of phenomenology, unlike ethnography, is to describe, rather than explain. It is important here to note that most researchers using a phenomenological approach do explain their findings as integral to undertaking research with a purpose. We will return to this later.

Pure phenomenological research is free from hypotheses and preconceptions. Husserl (1970) (considered the father of phenomenology) talks about the concept of the 'life world' as a key concept and focus of investigation for phenomenology, where the life world comprises the world of objects around us as we perceive them and our experience of our self, body and relationships. Life world is the world that is lived and experienced and takes place before we think about it or put it into language, i.e. before we have time to reflect on it. Merleau-Ponty (1962), another key figure in the development of phenomenology explains, 'man is in the world and only in that world does he know himself' (p. 10).

Box 2.4

Dyson *et al*. (2008) used a phenomenological approach to investigate the lived experiences of South Asian nursing students on pre-registration programmes in a UK university. Using this approach enabled the researchers to describe the world of the student in the particular context of being South Asian. The researchers came to know the world as lived by the student and were able to make recommendations for nurse educators in relation to supporting students from particular ethnic groups as they attempt to traverse an essentially ethnocentric curriculum.

There are numerous variants of phenomenological philosophy, for example *hermeneutic phenomenology*, which highlights the researchers role and interpretations in the research; heuristic phenomenology, which highlights the place of self-reflection in producing a creative account of the participant's lived experience; and relational research approaches, where attention is paid to the researcher's own journey (Finlay, 2008). The particular approach taken to conducting phenomenological research depends on the researcher's philosophical values, theoretical position and methodological preferences. However, broadly speaking phenomenology is flexible and allows for a wide range of investigations into issues in health and social care.

Finlay's (2008) features of phenomenological research are useful in helping us recognise phenomenological research:

- Phenomenology asks what this kind of experience is like.
- What does this experience mean?

- Phenomenological researchers help participants to express their world as directly as possible.
- Phenomenological researchers assist participants to reveal the dimensions of the lived world, so that the lived world is revealed.
- Meanings uncovered by the researcher emerge out of the way the researcher poses the questions. In particular, the researcher brackets or suspends previously held assumptions about the phenomenon in order to be open to the phenomenon as it appears.
- The researcher aims to be open and to see the world as the participant sees it.

Box 2.5

Barker (2010) carried out a study for a PhD thesis entitled 'The Midwife's Coracle: a phenomenological study of midwives' experiences of emotionally supporting motherhood' used a Husserlian phenomenological design. Unstructured interviews were conducted with eight community midwives in order to explore their experiences of providing emotional support to women who were becoming mothers. Barker (2010) was able to develop a general structure along with four constituents; 'tipping the balance to showing emotionally supportive care', 'showing emotionally supportive care', 'struggles in showing emotionally supportive care' and 'emotional experiences'. The descriptions of experiences shared by the midwives led to an understanding that emotional support is a special type of care. Barker, by using a phenomenological approach, was able to conclude that midwifery needs to consider how midwives might manage their 'with woman' care within health and social care services.

In summary, most research in the field of health and social care is not phenomenological in the true sense of the word. Researchers in health and social care more often than not use issues of concern for practitioners as their starting point. By this, I mean that the researchers already have a preconceived idea, if not a hypothesis, about the phenomenon under investigation. Very few researchers in health and social care do not take a view on what is happening in their field of practice. As such, it is usually the methods of data collection that are phenomenological, rather than the overall philosophical approach to the research. Nonetheless, phenomenological methods of data collection are extremely effective in prioritising and centralising the perspectives or voices of those affected by a given situation. In cases where these voices are marginalised (for example in a minority group or under-represented group), phenomenology, with its focus on the experiences and perceptions of the individuals concerned, can be extremely powerful in challenging the assumptions on which many structures in health and social care are founded.

Phenomenological research is done with relatively small numbers of participants, as is the case with all qualitative research where size does not matter. However, the ability of the research to add to the body of evidence about a particular phenomenon may be limited when small numbers of participants are included. In pure phenomenology, this does not matter, as the point is to describe the phenomenon from the individual's perspective and not necessarily to infer from the study to the broader population. However, in research in health and social care the point is often to make recommendations for future practice. Therefore, while phenomenological research can be robust in uncovering factors and their influence on individual cases it needs to be tentative in suggesting their extent in relation to the wider population from which the participants are drawn (Lester, 1999). This is a feature of all qualitative research and involves a move away from the concept of generalisability of research findings to a more appropriate discussion of transferability of research findings. We will consider this is more detail in a later chapter.

Grounded theory

Grounded theory is a particular approach to qualitative enquiry, which puts constant comparison of data at its heart. Barney Glaser and Anselm Strauss originally developed the method in 1967. In grounded theory the process begins with a research situation whereby the task of the researcher is to understand the roles of the players/actors in that situation. Data are collected from observations, conversations and/or interviews. Data from interviews (or other data) are compared to interviews (or other data), and data from observations (or other data) are compared to observations (or other data). After each episode of data collection, the researcher engages in a process of note taking as issues emerge.

Constant comparison is central to the process and theory tends to emerge quickly. The results of the comparisons of the note taking, written as codes, help the researchers to formulate categories and sub-categories, very much like themes and sub-themes. As this process of coding proceeds, the researcher begins to develop theoretical propositions, for example about links between categories or about a core category or one which is central to the study. The links between categories, sub-categories and core categories provide the theory. A key feature of grounded theory is the notes the researchers write to themselves, which act as memos. As the data collection and coding proceed, the notes and memos build up.

In grounded theory, the sample is added to theoretically. This is a purposive approach (we will look at this in more detail later), which increases the diversity of the sample by allowing the researcher to look for different properties. For example, if a core category becomes saturated with data, the researcher ceases data collection from this sample and moves on to the next category or sub-category. Data collection continues, increasing the sample as necessary until no new data emerges. When the process is complete, i.e. all categories and sub-categories are saturated, the researcher can move to the next step, which is sorting, whereby all memos (notes to self) accumulated are grouped in the order that best allows theory to become clear.

In grounded theory, literature is accessed as part of the process of data collection, coding, note taking and memo writing, and not generally undertaken as a predetermined search before data collection commences. This method allows literature to be accessed as necessary or as the need arises from emerging theory, which is grounded in the data. Glaser saw this as key to the method and argued that most research, including qualitative methodology is actually hypothesis testing.

Box 2.6

Kirkham and Stapleton (2000) adopted an ethnographic design for their study looking at midwives' support needs as childbirth changes, but used a grounded theory approach to data analysis. The researchers were of the view that grounded theory 'allows for the emergence and continual evolution of theoretical frameworks in synchrony with the actual research' (p. 466). Grounded theory accommodates a change within the interview format as the analysis develops. By asking the respondents different questions and allowing participants to address aspects or issues of importance to them the researchers were able to constantly explore categories, with some categories subsequently collapsed or merged, while others appeared.

The examples provided show how grounded theory allows ideas to emerge out of data, rather than existing prior to data collection, with the consequence that pre-existing or preformed views might influence theory development. In essence, theory is allowed to develop and build from the ground up, so to speak.

Dick (2005) provides a useful framework for identifying the essential steps in the process of grounded theory:

- The aim of grounded theory is to discover the theory implicit in the data.
- Grounded theory does not test a hypothesis.
- Grounded theory sets out to find what theory accounts for the research situation as it is.
- Data collection, note-taking, coding and memoing occur simultaneously.
- Sorting occurs when all categories are saturated.

Box 2.7

Toscano (2007), a nurse researcher in the USA, used grounded theory to investigate female adolescents' dating experiences and factors influencing safety. Twenty female adolescents aged between 15 and 18 were interviewed for her study, which aimed to describe the nature and characteristics of the dating relationships of adolescents females, including any experiences of abuse.

Toscano describes the process of data analysis:

Field notes of observations, emerging categories, relationships or theories were recorded manually during interviews, followed by a review of the audiotape recordings and field notes before subsequent interviews. Concepts formed from interview data were clarifed and converged with responses from participants. Data were transcribed and microanalysis was used to generate initial categories using open codes. Axial coding consisted of relating these initial categories back to their subcategories. Relational statements, grounded in the data, were connected using memos created during data analysis. Categories became saturated and concepts were fully defined. As categories emerged and evolved from the data, relationships between the categories were investigated via systematic comparison. Theoretical and operational notes directed the next step in the research process to finalize the theory (p. 3).

- Writing occurs after sorting.
- Theory is emergent – discovered in the data.

In summary, grounded theory is an emergent method. By this, we mean data collection begins as soon as a research situation arises and not at a later point, with literature being accessed as it becomes relevant. Glaser (1978) suggests that an alternative approach is to read broadly as a background to the research rather than reading the literature most closely associated with the subject of the research, as the latter approach may constrain coding and memoing. When using grounded theory the researcher carefully seeks disconfirming evidence as theory develops. In so doing, the grounded theorist is responsive to the data and draws on relevant literature as a simultaneous part of the research process.

Action research

Action research is fundamentally a research method aimed at changing practice. Action research works with practitioners and/or community members. Research findings, used immediately, continually develop and change practice. Action research undertaken *with* participants, rather than *to* them, always involves a collaborative and partnership approach to collecting data.

Action research is often credited to Kurt Lewin, a Prussian psychologist who later emigrated to the USA and worked mostly in the field of group dynamics. Lewin developed the concept of 'rational social management', which sought to combine experimental approaches with social action. Lewin believed in proceeding in a spiral of steps, each one composed of a circle of planning, action and fact finding about the result of the action. This approach characterises action research as we have come to know it and is an extremely powerful means of collaborating with practitioners to bring about positive change.

It should be noted that for action research to achieve its intended aim to 'improve and involve' (Carr and Kemmis, 1986, p. 165), equal partnership, whereby practitioners are deemed co-researchers, is essential. This partnership will usually see practitioners collecting data about their situation, finding strategies to solve the problem and converting the strategies into action (Holloway, 1997). The original researcher or person outside the practice arena may act as a catalyst for change and facilitate analysis of the situation by the practitioners, who are then empowered to instigate the necessary changes.

Action research involves the steps of planning, acting, observing/evaluating and reflecting, and these steps are integral to the design of the research and are taken with full participation of all stakeholders in the research. Figure 2.1 (overleaf) shows how the steps form a continuous process of planning, acting, observing/evaluating and reflecting to ensure that each action or change can be addressed if it does not meet the needs of those who will be affected by it.

In recent years, action research has come to be used to empower disenfranchised groups and to challenge the social structures that create such power imbalances. Action research when used in this way is known as participa-

Box 2.8

Wallis and Tyson (2003) wished to improve the nursing management of patients in a Haematology/Oncology day unit. Their action research approach commenced with a series of meetings involving day unit staff as a means of exploring and critically examining the nature and scope of problems with practice. Three phases of the action research process were undertaken, with each phase involving processes of observation, reflection, action and evaluation. Data were gathered from staff meetings, examination of incident reports, patients' complaints and observations of clinical staff, subsequently exposing serious problems with patient waiting times within the unit and variability in staff workload.

The observation phase enabled a team of staff to develop a chemotherapy protocol which could be used to plan patient care and to allocate staff more appropriately. The time required for administration of the protocol at each patient visit was recorded along with the factors which variously affected administration, for example pharmacy time, setup time for the chemotherapy, and the actual time taken for each clinical health assessment. Using action research in this way enabled the team to move from simple development of the protocol to the more complex development of an appointment system which reflected the actual time required to use the protocol. Over time, as the team implemented the protocol and appointment system, the process of reflection and evaluation exposed additional concerns (for example waiting rooms being full throughout the day, with obvious implications for patients). The action research cycle was revisited to improve the patient appointment booking system and staff allocation.

tory action research, and is premised on the notion of co-researchers working together as equal partners trying out various actions, observing those actions, and evaluating and reflecting on the effectiveness of the actions in improving practice. This process allows the co-researchers to analyse the situation they are in, to develop solutions to real-world problems, and to become empowered to bring about positive change. In situations where professional practice is dictated by polices outside the control or influence of the practitioners themselves, participatory action research is a powerful research method to provide the evidence base for changing practice. However, it should be noted that the problems must be those identified by the practitioners themselves and not suggested or imposed by the organisation. In cases where the issues are not those identified by practitioners, then true participatory action research is not undertaken and the method is used to maintain the status quo or to instigate change against the wishes of the practitioners.

Wadsworth (1998) provides us with an explanation of participatory action research:

■ Participatory action research consciously problematises an existing action or practice and defines who is problematising it and why.
■ Participatory action research consciously names the problem, raises questions about the problem and focuses on the need to answer the question.
■ Participatory action research is planned and deliberate about commencing the process of inquiry and consciously considers all those who need to be involved in the inquiry.
■ Participatory action research is systematic and rigorous in its efforts to get answers to the problematic action or practice.

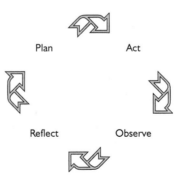

Plan   Act

Reflect   Observe

Figure 2.1 Steps in action research.

- Participatory action research carefully documents and records each action taken to address the problem and what people think about each action taken, in ways that are relevant and meaningful to all interested parties.
- Participatory action research is intensive, comprehensive and cautious, before jumping to conclusions.
- Participatory action research attempts to develop deep understanding and more useful and powerful theory about the problem in order to improve action or practice.
- Changing action or practice is fundamental to participatory action research and is followed by further participatory action research to investigate the changed action or practice.

In summary, action research (and participatory action research in particular) considers it critical to the success of the inquiry that the question posed in the first place is one that is relevant and useful to those affected. Participatory action research considers where the problems have come from and insists that new actions or practices arising from the inquiry are tested in action. In participatory action research a cyclical, rather than a linear, model is used, which starts with reflection on action, and proceeds to new action, which is then further researched until all those participating in delivering the service agree best practice.

Feminist research

Feminist research studies the social content of women's lives from a stand-point that essentially views society as patriarchal and male-dominated. The aim of feminist research is to enlighten society about the taken-for-granted sexist practices and gender blindness of governments and most community practices that have led to the displacement of women, ignoring of women and often the silencing of women. Feminist research is research by women for women, with the intention of making women visible, raising their consciousness and empowering them (Holloway, 1997).

Feminist research traces its roots in feminist theory. Cott (1987) delineates modern feminist theory from its antecedents, particularly the struggle for suffrage. A distinction may be drawn between the women's movement prior to suffrage, which was primarily about the woman as a universal entity, and the post-suffrage movement, which was more concerned with social differentiation. In recent times feminist theory has dealt with issues such as women's condition as a social construct, gender identity and relationships within and between genders. Feminist research is based on this body of critical theory built over time. As you would expect, feminist research is, by its very nature, critical and emancipatory, perceiving reality, science and research in this context.

The methods employed by feminist researchers generally fit best with the interpretivist paradigm, as the assumption underpinning feminist research is the world as a socially constructed place. However, feminists do and have used quantitative methods if the nature of the inquiry requires them to do so. This recourse to a mixed methods approach in feminist research has caused some consternation for feminists, who believe that the true feminist position rejects any form of positivism. For postmodern feminist researchers a more liberal approach allows for and requires that the methods of data collection be dictated by the inquiry itself. All feminist research seeks to be value-free and to place the interests of women as central to its endeavour.

Feminist research lends itself particularly well to issues of concerns for midwives by allowing women's and midwives' voices to be heard.

Sarantakos (2005) provides us with a clear and concise guide to the principles on which feminist research is premised:

- Women have been marginalised.
- Male superiority is perpetuated despite policies, assurances and political promises.

Box 2.9

Keating and Fleming (2009) used a feminist perspective to explore the experiences of midwives of facilitating normal birth in an obstetric-led unit. The researchers utilised a feminist approach within semi-structured interviews with midwives working on the unit. The midwives' narratives related to the concepts of patriarchy: hierarchical thinking, power and prestige, and a logic of domination. The researchers were able to identify a number of reasons why midwives find it difficult to facilitate normal birth in an obstetric-led unit and recommended supportive management structures if midwives are to become confident practitioners of normal birth.

- That males and females are considered physically and emotionally different, with men being considered superior.
- That there is still a long way to go to establish gender equality.
- That the relationship between researcher and researched requires serious reconsideration.

In summary, feminist research takes as its focus the experiences and perceptions of women. As Holloway (1997) succinctly puts it, feminist approaches do not prescribe methods of analysing research but suggest ways of thinking about it. However, the commonality in all feminist research is the positioning of the 'feminine' as central, with the intention of making the often invisible woman visible. While some feminist researchers argue for a distinct and separate feminist research methodology, others take a more liberal view and argue that feminist research is research that aims to change the status of women in society, to redress the balance, to study women. In this sense, feminist research, irrespective of methodology, is research conducted on women, for women and by women.

Narrative research

Narrative research epitomises the qualitative approach to research perhaps more than any other methodology, being naturalistic, phenomenological, ethnographic and inherently subjective (Polkinghorne, 1988). The core of narrative research is relativism, rather than absolute truths; in other words there is an acceptance on the part of the researcher of the existence of more than one reality or truth. This fundamental aspect of narrative research makes it the ideal approach for researchers in health and social care who wish to understand the life stories of individuals experiencing physical and psychological ill health, and indeed for all research that seeks to understand the life trajectories of individuals.

Consider the case of asylum seekers fleeing from countries where life is made unsustainable by governments hostile to dissent of any kind. On arrival in the UK asylum seekers are detained until the Home Office hears their cases, which can take up to two years (Cleave, 2009). Narrative research is especially sensitive to the unique characteristics of human existence and is therefore ideal for research that aims to come as close as possible to the meaning of subjective experience. Narrative research enables social scientists to study people rather than variables.

Box 2.10

Dyson (2005) examined the life experiences of Zimbabwean nursing students studying in the UK. A narrative approach was employed to understand the life histories of students leaving their homeland to live, study and (in most cases) work in another country, and the meaning they attributed to these experiences. A narrative approach allowed stories to be told in the students' voice. For the first time since arriving in the UK students were able to share previously untold aspects of their lives, including what it is like to leave their country of birth, find accommodation, and begin studying in the UK, at the same time as remitting monies home for families who needed help and support to remain in Zimbabwe.

Narrative research has the potential to draw attention to the voices of marginalised people, often silenced through circumstances beyond their control. In this sense, narrative research is both powerful and sensitive in ways that other methodologies are not.

Narrative research is not without its challenges. The first of these is the amount of material generated from narrative interviewing. Respondents, invited to tell their stories in their own words, and in their own context, often include a personal time frame. Narrative interviewing requires the respondent to cede the floor to the teller in other words to step back and allow the respondent to take over the conversation. This is essential, as story telling is the focus of the research and the story itself is the object of the investigation.

The second challenge lies with the analysis. Narrative is subtle, complex and difficult to interpret (Riessman, 1993). Accounts of stories told by respondents are often multifaceted, and can be at odds with the researcher's firmly held views of the social world, including what the researcher thinks they know of the world of the respondent. To complicate matters further, notions of reality and identity are constructions that take place on different levels, within a certain context and in a certain language, and much can be lost in translation.

Nevertheless, in spite of the challenges of using a narrative approach people do live the events and affairs of their lives in a storied way. What we think we know of another's life is more often than not far removed from the 'truth' as that person experiences it. Narrative research allows us to make sense of experiences by casting them in a narrative and gives an insight into the intensely human realm of value (Riessman, 1993).

Riessman (1993) suggests that all narrative research has the following characteristics:

- It aims to study people by listening.
- The act of listening implies sensitivity to the unique characteristics of human existence.
- It is guided by a core of consensus regarding facts, traits and processes, about which different subjective accounts agree.
- It aims towards novel observational experience.
- It creates new views about man's social world.

Narratives are stories told by individuals about their condition, work or lives. Narratives have existed for centuries in the forms of diaries, oral histories or travellers' tales. The systematic collection of stories, whatever their form, is known as narrative research. The narrative approach, although not without its challenges, is especially useful for studying transformations and transitions in individuals' lives and is therefore a powerful methodological approach for researching aspects of health and illness (Holloway, 1997).

Conclusion

In conclusion, in this chapter we considered what we mean by qualitative research. Qualitative research, founded on the belief that the social world, or world inhabited by individuals, can only be known by asking questions of individuals about how they are affected by a particular issue: what impact the issue has on their lives, what sense they make of the issue, and how they would change their situation if they could. Qualitative research is not interested in knowing the extent of the issue or the range of issues. In this sense, qualitative research fits within the interpretivist paradigm, which focuses on human beings and the way they interpret and make sense of reality.

We then considered a number of approaches to conducting qualitative research, including ethnography, phenomenology, grounded theory, action research, feminist research and narrative research. These approaches are not exhaustive, but will enable you to recognise qualitative research and the different approaches that qualitative researchers take to their work, based on the kinds of questions they seek to answer. In the next chapter, we look at strategies for selecting participants, and methods for collecting and analysing data in qualitative research.

Further reading

Bryman, A. (2001) *Social Research Methods*. Oxford University Press, Oxford.

Cluett, E. R. and Bluff, R. (eds.) (2006) *Principles and Practice of Research in Midwifery*, 2nd edn. Elsevier, Oxford.

Holloway, I. (1997) *Basic Concepts for Qualitative Research*. Blackwell Science, Oxford.

Hughes, C. (2002) *Key Concepts in Feminist Theory and Research*. Sage, London.

Parahoo, K. (2006) *Nursing Research. Principles, Process and Issues*, 2nd edn. Palgrave MacMillan, Basingstoke.

CHAPTER 3

Qualitative research: data collection and analysis

Introduction

Methods for data collection employed in qualitative research may vary. However, the most commonly used approaches include direct observation, interviews or focus groups, and analysis of texts and documents and of recorded speech, such as video and audio tapes (Pope and Mays, 2000). The key feature of all these data collection techniques is the emphasis on the actual events and the verbalisation of events by those experiencing them, rather than on numbers. In this sense, as Pope and Mays (2000, p. 7) suggest, these methods (at least on one level) are those we use in everyday situations as we try to make sense of the world – 'we watch what is going on, ask questions of each other and try to comprehend the social world we live in'.

Before we look in detail at methods of data collection in qualitative research it is important to understand what we mean by *population* and *sample*:

Research population: all the individuals with the characteristics one wishes to understand

Research sample: a subset of the population with the characteristics of the population, who represent the population

The research question determines the population and subsequent sample for data collection and needs to be considered before methods for data collection and subsequent analysis are chosen. Examples of population and samples in nursing and midwifery research are given below.

- *Nursing*: stroke survivors; young adults with mental health diagnoses; patients undergoing chemotherapy
- *Midwifery*: pregnant women; women diagnosed with post-natal depression; women who choose home birth

Sampling in qualitative research

In qualitative research, it is not possible to collect data from everyone in a given community or population due to the methods used, for example interviews and focus groups. Therefore, qualitative researchers choose a sample or subset of a population using a specific strategy to ensure that the sample is representative of the population they wish to study. The sampling strategy is guided by the research question, the research aims and objectives and to a certain extent by the resources available to the researcher. There are three main sampling strategies: purposive, quota and snowball.

Purposive sampling

Purposive sampling is the most common strategy open to qualitative researchers and occurs when participants are grouped according to pre-set criteria relevant to the research study. In some research studies, it is important to the research question to ensure that the participants in the research exhibit the characteristics the researchers wish to investigate. In other studies there are no essential criteria, as the research question is broad rather than specific. The more specific the research question, the more specific the criteria for inclusion and exclusion from the study.

In purposive sampling, the number of participants may be determined by resources available to the researcher or the point at which theoretical saturation occurs. By this, we mean the point in data collection where new data no longer bring additional insights to the research question.

Purposive sampling is sometimes referred to as judgemental, selective or subjective. The goal is *not* to select participants randomly from a population to create a sample, in order to make generalisations from your sample to the rest of the population once the research has been carried out. The goal of purposive

Table 3.1 Research questions, populations and samples.

Research question	Population	Sample characteristics
Factors influencing smoking behaviour in pregnancy	Pregnant mothers	Pregnant mothers who smoke during pregnancy
An exploration of the experiences of infertile women undergoing fertility treatment	Infertile women	Infertile women undergoing fertility treatments
An exploration of Zimbabwean nursing students experiences in a UK university	Nursing students at the university	Zimbabwean nursing students

sampling *is* to concentrate on those characteristics or features of the population that are of interest to you, the researcher, in relation to your research question.

Table 3.1 gives examples of where purposive sampling might be used in nursing and midwifery research.

Quota sampling

Quota sampling is a type of purposive sampling. However, the size and characteristics are determined prior to data collection at the stage of study design. Characteristics might include students studying a particular programme, in a particular year of study, or of a particular age, gender or ethnicity. Setting criteria in this way allows the qualitative researcher to choose participants who are most likely to have an insight into the focus of the study. The researcher determines the criteria, then goes into the community or population of interest and collects data from that group until the quota is reached.

Purposive and quota sampling depend on the identification of participants based on selected criteria. Quota sampling can be problematic as a result of its unreliability, in that the researcher decides beforehand how many participants in a given category are selected. When the quota is reached the sampling ceases, which means not everyone will get a chance of being selected. Quota sampling is useful when time is limited. An alternative to quota sampling, which

Box 3.1

A researcher is interested in the attitudes of nursing students from different religions towards termination of pregnancy. In a given part of the UK a random sample might miss Muslim nursing students because there are not many in that particular area of the country. To ensure inclusion of Muslim nursing students in the study, the research could set a quota for the sample. The sample will not then be representative of the actual proportion of Muslim nursing students in the population (which may have an effect on generalisation). However, the *quota* guarantees that the views of Muslim student nurses are represented in the study.

addresses the problem of reliability and fairness, involves stratification of the sample. In stratified sampling, subsets of the population are created whereby each subset has a common characteristic (for example trimester of pregnancy or chemotherapy treatment regime). An example of quota sampling is given below.

Snowball sampling

Snowball sampling is also a type of purposive sampling. However, this strategy depends on respondents identifying individuals known to them who might be interested in participating in the research. Snowball sampling is particularly useful with hard to reach groups. However, it does depend on identifying initial respondents who then 'get the snowball rolling'. Snowball sampling is sometimes referred to as chain sampling, chain-referral sampling or referral sampling. When using snowball sampling the researcher needs to be mindful of the problem of bias, in that the technique itself reduces the likelihood that the sample will represent a good cross-section of the population. Sample members are often not selected by the researchers from a sampling frame, but are referred to the researcher by existing participants in the research – often friends or acquaintances. The issue of bias is of obvious concern and researchers need to be clear as to why this type of sampling is used, as opposed to another sampling strategy. 'Hard to reach' groups may be accessed through social networks and lend themselves to snowball sampling strategies. Some examples of hard to reach groups are provided below.

- Users of drugs in pregnancy
- Individuals with undisclosed mental health issues at work
- Teenagers engaging in online chat rooms
- Women who have given children up for adoption
- Infertile Asian women

It is worth noting that in qualitative work the researcher is not rigidly bound by the original sampling strategy. It is acceptable to mix sampling strategies or to refine the strategy depending on the progress of data collection. This flexibility allows sampling for later stages of the research to be guided by earlier findings.

Collecting qualitative data

Direct observation

In qualitative research, where it is important that the researcher is immersed in the area to be studied, data are collected through observing people in their own environments. This might be the observation of a particular occupational group, such as nurses, doctors or physiotherapists, or observations of patients in healthcare settings. The aim is for the researcher to develop an understanding of the values and beliefs held by the population under investigation.

Participant observation

In direct observation information can be collected by a *participant* observer, for example a nurse undertaking normal duties may observe the processes going on in a care setting and collect data during the course of a shift, or a midwife might observe the promotion of breast feeding by midwives on a post-natal ward in the course of a routine day. Alternatively, a *non-participant* observer, for example a non-nurse, may observe nurses at work and collect data during the course of a shift, or a non-midwife might observe midwives engaged in promoting breast feeding in the immediate post-natal period. Both approaches are legitimate and choice depends on the research question.

Take, for example, a research study where the aim is to understand the interpersonal relationships between nurse managers and ward staff, over the course of a working day. Here it would be difficult for a researcher who is not part of the nursing team to have complete access to the full range of activities that make up the nursing 'work', for example day-to-day care, team meetings, ward rounds and handovers. It is unlikely that a non-participant observer would come to understand how interpersonal relationships between members of the nursing team play out in the day-to-day life of the ward. On the other hand, a participant observer, for example a member of the nursing team, would naturally participate in a range of nursing activities where interpersonal relationships are a key feature of the working day. Thus, the observer would be able to collect the data required to answer the research question in a way that enhances the trustworthiness of the findings. Similarly, it might be extremely difficult for a non-midwife to observe and understand a midwife's approach to promoting breast feeding with a young mother without a detailed understanding of the women's thoughts and feelings on breast feeding.

Participant observation in qualitative research is viewed on a continuum, whereby at the extreme the observer is completely immersed in the area under investigation. In this case, the observer is usually a natural participant and may be observing a situation of which they are naturally a part. At the other end of the continuum the researcher may be quite external to the observation, in some cases observing through the medium of television, video conferencing or other media. In most cases participant observation falls somewhere in between.

James Key (1997) identifies five types of participant observation (external, passive, balanced, active and total), all of which allow for more or less interaction with the participants. However, each type relies on systematically seeking out and organising data, the concern being with what is studied, rather than focusing on achieving a situationally defined goal. The participant observer keeps detailed records of everything that occurs, including those things normally taken for granted or naturally occurring in the setting. In addition, the participant observer periodically removes himself or herself from the situation in order to review data collected from a neutral position, monitors observations constantly, and records data in an unbiased way.

Non-participant observation

In non-participant observation, the researcher watches the subjects of the study with their consent, but takes no active part in the situation. A key consideration here is that most people, on knowing they are being observed, will usually act differently to some degree, a phenomenon known as the 'Hawthorn Effect', a termed coined to describe the behaviour-modifying effects of being the subject of social investigation, rather than the context of the investigation. One way in which researchers can mitigate the Hawthorn Effect is to observe similar situations over time, although this has obvious resource implications. Alternatively, video recording equipment may be used, although this only limits the Hawthorn Effect and does not eradicate it.

Interviews

Interviews allow for the collection of detailed data from the population studied, which can be analysed in detail later. Interviews can take place in any setting, and are usually located at a place convenient to respondents and researchers, i.e. a mutually agreed time and location. Quantitative data collection techniques such as questionnaires may include open-ended questions and facilitate data collection from large numbers of respondents in a way not permitted by interviews. However, the potential of the interview to permit probing of issues of interest to the researcher that may pre-exist the interview or occur as the interview proceeds remains one of the key benefits. Interviews can be in-depth, structured, semi-structured, informal or formal.

In-depth interviews

In-depth interviews are usually conducted at a venue convenient to the respondent or mutually agreed by respondent and researcher. The key to successful interviewing is for the respondent to feel at ease and for the researcher to be well prepared before the interview begins, which may require equipment for audio recording the interview, and an interview schedule, either structured or semi-structured. This necessitates forward planning in order that time is used effectively and that the data collected are meaningful and appropriate for the study.

In-depth interviews allow the researcher to gather data rich in depth and detail. Unlike when using a survey in quantitative research, the researcher rarely has a predetermined set of questions, as the objective of in-depth interviewing is to encourage the respondent to express their views at length in their own words. As we saw in the previous chapter, qualitative research requires the researcher to allow the human participants to guide, control and direct the inquiry. Therefore the skill of the in-depth interviewer is in facilitation, rather than controlling the process of data collection.

In-depth interviewing leads to particular challenges for the researcher, not least in ensuring that the data collected are appropriate to the study. For this reason, the researcher may choose a structured or semi-structured approach.

Structured interviews

A structured approach to interviewing is appropriate when the interviewer is familiar with the subject matter of the research. Although not a survey as such, a formalised questionnaire can be used to direct the interview along a predetermined set of questions. The respondent is able to answer the questions in their own words. However, the degree of flexibility is far less than in semi-structured interviews. The main advantage of structured interviews is their ability to allow sequencing of questions, which subsequently facilitates sequenced analysis.

This approach would not lend itself to qualitative methodologies where it is imperative to give complete freedom to the respondent, for example in narrative research. However when using grounded theory interviewers may use a progressive focusing technique, whereby the researcher asks the respondents a predetermined set of questions that have arisen from prior data collection. Although answered in the respondent's own words, this focused or structured approach allows the researcher to pursue ideas and questions grounded in the data (Holloway, 1997).

A further reason for choosing a structured approach is when the researcher wishes to undertake a large number of interviews but prefers not to undertake a survey, which generally lends itself to quantitative research. In this case, a structured approach may enable the more effective use of resources, with the interview guided in terms of questions and available time by the use of a structured interview guide.

Semi-structured interviews

Semi-structured interviews use an open framework. The key is to facilitate a focused two-way conversation between researcher and respondent. The usual method in this approach is to start the interview with a general question and move to specific questions as the interview progresses. The specific questions may or may not arise out of the previous questions, i.e. as a response to answers given earlier. A semi-structured approach is useful, much the same as a structured approach when time is of the essence and the emphasis is on making best use of available time and for effective use of resources, such as the availability of the respondent, researcher and facilities for conducting the interview.

A semi-structured approach allows consideration of relevant topics prior to the interview. A greater degree of flexibility than with a structured approach allows opportunities for deviation from the prescribed topic. In semi-structured interviewing, while the topic is identified beforehand, the majority of questions are created during the interview itself. An interview guide used in semi-structured interviewing is for framing the interview, and not for directing it *per se*.

Focus groups

Focus groups are a form of group interviewing with a subtle difference, in that the key feature of the focus group is the interaction that takes place between the respondents. Unlike group interviews, whereby the researcher may interview a number of respondents at the same time with the emphasis on questions and responses between researcher and recipients, the focus group relies on interaction within the group prompted by topics supplied by the researcher (Morgan, 1997). The reason for choosing focus groups to collect qualitative data rather than other methods, such as one-to-one interviews, group interviews or questionnaire surveys, lies in the ability of the focus group to draw out the attitudes, feelings and beliefs that individuals may hold on a given issue through the process of social interaction.

The emotional processes and multiplicity of views elicited through group interaction are a powerful tool for the qualitative researcher. However, the very nature of the focus group and its capacity to draw on respondents' core attitudes, values and beliefs require a skilled interviewer and thoughtful preparation before undertaking this method of data collection.

Focus group interviewing requires the researcher to have an interview guide prior to beginning the focus group. It is important for the researcher to ensure that the focus group achieves its aim, which is to enable all participants to discuss and comment on the issue fully while avoiding the tendency for any one participant to take over and dominate proceedings to the detriment of other voices. In this sense, an individual interview may be easier to control than a focus group in which participants may take control. A well-thought-out interview guide enables the researcher to draw participants back to the topic at hand and to remain in control of the process should the topic move too far from the focus of the research.

Focus groups can be extremely useful for exploring dynamics between groups, where the researcher is interested in power relationships between decision-makers and professionals, or where everyday use of language and culture of particular groups is of interest (Morgan, 1997).

Focus groups are particularly useful in a participatory action research context, in that they provide an opportunity for participants to be involved in the decision-making process, to be valued as experts, and to be given the chance to work collaboratively with researchers; all key features of participatory action research. In this sense, focus groups can be extremely empowering.

However, the researcher choosing to use the focus group technique needs to be mindful that some participants may be less articulate, less confident and often more introverted than others. In these situations some participants may find the focus group intimidating and consequently not as empowering an experience as for other members of the group.

From a practical point of view, focus groups need time to set up. Efforts need to be taken to ensure a representative sample within the group, which may be difficult if respondents feel themselves to be inarticulate, lacking in confidence or to have communication difficulties. If this is the case then rather than compromise the research and alienate respondents who may have an important contribution to make, other methods, such as individual interviews, should be considered.

The final point to make about focus groups (and group interviews for that matter) is that they can never be completely confidential or anonymous, as information is shared with the group. Participants in the focus group should be made aware of this before consenting to take part. The researcher, for their part, should set ground rules for all participants in the focus group, which addresses the ethical issue of confidentiality. Although information is shared within the group and will be used for the purposes of the research, participants must be encouraged not to share information outside the group. The researcher must anonymise all data collected from the group to ensure that no individual participant can be identified.

Documentary sources

In some cases it is not possible to gather data from participants, because a particular group may be inaccessible, no longer viable or in existence, unwilling to participate, or have been overused in research. In certain situations, to subject groups or individuals to further research would be traumatic (for example victims of crime, abuse or extreme trauma). In these situations, it may be possible to collect data or supplement existing data with documentary evidence.

A number of different sources are available as documentary evidence, and these can be central or peripheral to the study. Documentary evidence may derive from private or public material (for example minutes of private meetings, legal documents or confidential reports) or documents in the public domain, such as textbooks, academic journals and other archived materials. A distinction is drawn between the formal or informal nature of documentary sources. For example, diaries, journals and memoirs may constitute informal sources, as opposed to more formal documents such as official reports.

'Documentary' is sometimes applied to data collected from oral narratives and certain non-textual objects, such as works of art (Sim and Wright, 2000). Documentary sources used retrospectively are generally considered as secondary research, in that the data were created or assembled before the current research was carried out, whereas data not specifically created for the research is deemed a secondary source on which primary research is being carried out. As such, primary data are always subject to primary analysis, whereas secondary data may be subject to either primary or secondary analysis.

Drawbacks

A criticism of the aforementioned qualitative methods of data collection (indeed of qualitative research in general) is that only small numbers of participants can be studied because the data collection methods are so labour-intensive. In addition, qualitative research is often criticised for being subject to researcher bias, difficulties in analysing qualitative data rigorously, and the lack of reproducibility and generalisability of the findings. We consider strategies for overcoming these difficulties next.

Qualitative data analysis

Qualitative data analysis is the process whereby we proceed from data collection to interpretation, explanation and understanding of the participants and situations of interest to us. In keeping with the philosophy underpinning qualitative research, where we are interested to know what a given situation or experience was like for the individual, the idea is to come to know someone's view of the world: how he or she came to that view and what meaning they attribute to their experience. For the majority of data collection in qualitative research, be it from interviews, focus groups, case study or role-play, the process of data analysis involves the key steps of coding and identifying themes (Lewins *et al.*, 2005). In discourse analysis or other forms of narrative research, identification of themes may not be required. Seidal (1998) likens qualitative data analysis to a jigsaw puzzle and uses the framework of noticing, collecting and thinking to structure the analysis of qualitative data.

Noticing

Noticing things in the data may initially begin with making observations, writing field notes, audio recording interviews and gathering documents, the point of which is to produce a record of the things we have noticed. Once the record is produced and subsequently focused on, further interesting things may be noticed in the data. As these interesting things are noticed, they are coded. Coding in the manner described here allows the data to be collected together. The researcher searches the collected data for types, words, sentences, phrases, patterns or wholes, with the aim of reconstructing the data into a meaningful or comprehensible account. Codes are used to pull together and categorise what would otherwise be confusing and unrelated accounts.

Collecting

Lewins *et al.* (2005) begin their guidelines on qualitative data analysis by considering what it means to write about the data collected. They suggest that what the researcher initially writes may contain some analytic ideas, in other words the process of analysis begins early. On the other hand, the researcher may simply summarise data, with the analytic process coming later. Whatever the approach, the point of writing is to organise the data into manageable parts in order that the identification of themes can begin. Coding the data is an essential part of this process.

Coding allows the application of labels to sections of the data that look as though they might belong to a theme. For example, in qualitative research undertaken with South Asian student nurses, collected from face-to-face interviews, we were interested to know of their experiences of studying an undergraduate nursing programme (Dyson *et al.*, 2008). The researchers read the interview transcripts and circled what seemed to be key words, phrases or events, writing short notes at the side of the circled text. This initial coding led to a list, part of which we show here:

- negotiation with family to leave home to study at university
- nursing as a positive career choice
- fear of failure
- perceptions of support from tutors at university
- career aspirations

As you can see, some parts of the list are simple descriptions of what the students said (for example fear of failure), whereas other parts are more analytical (for example nursing as a positive career choice). This list (abridged here) was used to 'mark up' the rest of the transcript and other transcripts in order that comparisons could be made. 'Negotiation to study' recurred across the transcripts and generated the theme: negotiated journeys.

Coding has been used in midwifery research by Kirkham and Stapleton (2000), who were interested to know how midwives described their support needs as childbirth changes. The researchers conducted 168 interviews with midwives from all grades and practice settings across six different midwifery sites. The researchers describe a process of selectively coding the interview transcripts before developing categories, which were then constantly explored in ongoing interviews and analysis, a method consistent with a grounded theory approach (Glaser and Strauss, 1967). Using coding to identify key words assists in the development of categories which are 'grounded' in the data.

A two-step process may be followed where basic coding is used to distinguish overall themes, followed by a more detailed interpretive coding, where specific patterns can be interpreted (Hay, 2005). The categories developed by

Kirkham and Stapleton (2000), following the initial coding process, are shown below.

- The culture of the NHS and the need for support
- Listening/being there
- Vulnerability and the need for protection
- Needs for advocacy and facilitation
- The danger of dependency
- Support and trust
- Enhancing midwives' confidence
- Midwives outside the NHS
- Support towards flexible and sustainable caring

Coding in qualitative research can be performed manually, for example by using coloured highlighter pens to differentiate between concepts – a method I've used myself – or by feeding key words into a qualitative software package (for example Atlas or NVivo). Computer packages will not analyse the data for you, but may make the process of coding and categorising less time-consuming.

Thinking

Once the process of collecting and sorting has been undertaken, the next step in qualitative data analysis is to think about the data. In the thinking stage the researcher is engaged in examining the collected account; the goal being to make sense out of what has been collected together, to look for patterns and relationships within and across collections and to make discoveries about the phenomena being studied.

Criticisms

There are, of course, some criticisms of the model of qualitative data analysis presented here, namely that the process of breaking down the data into small parts can destroy the totality of the philosophy as expressed by the interviewee. The very act of breaking down the data into its constituent parts can sometimes distort the analysis. A way round this is to work between two accounts or transcripts: a coded version and an intact version. In this way, the researcher can work back and forth between the parts and the whole. There are alternative ways of analysing qualitative data that do not involve the process of noticing (making notes and writing about the data), collecting (coding the data) and thinking (looking for patterns, identifying themes within and across the data). The model of noticing, collecting and thinking does run the risk of describing the codes but losing the phenomena. Nevertheless, it is an extremely useful and pragmatic approach to qualitative data analysis.

Computer-assisted qualitative data analysis

Qualitative research can produce large amounts of data in the form of interview or focus group transcripts, often running to many pages. With the advent of computer software packages, qualitative data analysis can be managed efficiently without losing the quality of the analysis. Computer-assisted qualitative data analysis allows not only the coding and retrieval of text, but also rapid searching through the transcripts that would ordinarily take the researcher an age to do – hence the cost-effectiveness of using computer-assisted qualitative data analysis. However, should this technology be used, the researcher must invest the time and effort to ensure they are familiar with the programme. Integral to this is an understanding of what the software can and cannot do. In general, computer-assisted qualitative data analysis, whichever package is used, provides the researcher with a workspace in which to work through information quickly and easily. Tools within the package assist in classifying, sorting and arranging data, which would otherwise be managed by hand. This frees time for exploring trends, finding meaning and arriving at answers. The computer assists the researcher with data management but does not *think* for the researcher.

Conclusion

In conclusion, we have considered strategies for identifying respondents in qualitative research, including purposive, quota and snowball techniques. We noted that qualitative researchers might draw on a mixture of approaches or refine the approach as data collection proceeds in order to achieve theoretical saturation. We then looked at techniques for collecting qualitative data, including observation, interviews, and focus groups. These techniques rely on the presence, to a greater or lesser extent, of participants in the research. We also considered analysis of texts and documents: a method available to qualitative researchers when collection of data from individuals is difficult or impossible. There are other methods of collecting qualitative data, for example diary methods (where the researcher or participant keeps a personal account of daily events, feelings, discussions and interactions); role play (where participants play a role or observe role play prior to rating behaviour) and case study (an in-depth study of one person, group or event).

Finally, we looked at qualitative data analysis, focusing in particular on Seidal's (1998) model of noticing, collecting and thinking. Within this model, we have looked at coding the data prior to identifying and organising into themes. Seidal's model allows more detailed approaches to qualitative data analysis to be carried out within its broad framework, including the constant comparative method and the extremely detailed method of qualitative data analysis used in grounded theory and described in the previous chapter. Criticisms and inherent risks of Seidal's approach to qualitative data analysis are noted, in particular that coding involves breaking the transcripts down into small parts, with the result that the integrity of the expressed account may be lost. One solution to this problem is to work back and forth between a coded account and an intact account. Finally, we considered the benefits and disadvantages afforded to qualitative data analysis in using computer-assisted packages. In the next chapter, we consider quality and ethics in qualitative research.

Further reading

Holloway, I. (ed.) (2005) *Qualitative Research in Health Care*. Open University Press, Berkshire.

Pope, C. and Mays, N. (eds.) (2006) *Qualitative Research in Health Care*, 3rd edn. Blackwell, Oxford.

Ritchie, J. (ed.) (2003) *Qualitative Research Practice: A Guide for Social Science Students and Researchers*. Sage, London.

Silverman, D. (2009) *Doing Qualitative Research*, 3rd edn. Sage, London.

CHAPTER 4

Qualitative research: quality and ethics

Introduction

So far in this book we have looked at research philosophies, methodologies, methods, data collection and analysis. We have learnt that qualitative research is concerned in the main with the systematic collection, ordering, description and interpretation of textual data generated from talk, observation or documentation. Qualitative research methods of data collection are many and varied, including interviewing, observation and documentary analysis. Whatever the method, the aim of qualitative research is, as Kitto *et al.* (2008) suggest, to explore the behaviour, processes of interaction, and the meaning, values and experiences of purposefully sampled individuals and groups in their natural context. Quantitative research, on the other hand, is concerned with the size or extent of a phenomenon. Data are collected and subjected to statistical tests, to allow prediction and generalisation to the broader population.

Given the difference in frameworks for data collection and analysis in qualitative and quantitative research, it is fair to suggest that considerations of quality should be approached differently. The conventional criteria of validity, reliability and generalisability as applied to quantitative research do not fit with qualitative research because the goal or aim is intrinsically different, as are the sampling strategies, including sample size. Consequently, the criteria of clarification and justification, procedural rigour, representativeness, interpretation, reflexivity and evaluative rigour, and transferability are used to ensure a comprehensive framework for addressing quality in qualitative research (Kitto *et al.*, 2008).

Clarification and justification

In Chapter 2 we looked at the research methodologies used in qualitative research, focusing in particular on ethnography, phenomenology, grounded theory, action research, narrative research and feminist research. In all these forms of research, clarity of purpose and how this is translated into the research aims and objectives is essential, and key to addressing the concern with quality in qualitative research. The qualitative researcher must pay attention to, and be able to demonstrate, a rigorous approach to determining the best fit between the research question, aims and objectives, and the chosen methodology and methods of data collection.

For example, if the aims of a research project are to understand from the perspectives of the respondents what it is like to live with a long-term condition, then an appropriate methodology may be phenomenology, given that phenomenology assists participants to reveal dimensions of the lived world so that the lived world is revealed. Alternatively, if a researcher wishes to understand cultural practice on a busy labour ward, and how midwives experience working in this multidisciplinary setting, then ethnography would provide a best fit as it allows the researcher to study respondents in their everyday context. This is not to say that only one approach or design will suffice, to the exclusion of all others. As discussed earlier, methodological blindness, where the researcher claims to have found the one true methodological position, limits the potential for qualitative research to enable respondents to tell their stories in their own words. Rather, the question is one of clarification and justification on the part of the researcher as to why a particular approach as opposed to an alternative. Thus, clarification (what is the research question) and justification (why this approach to the research design) are integral considerations for the qualitative researcher.

Procedural rigour

Procedural rigour in qualitative research refers to the transparency adopted by the researchers in reporting and recording each step in the research process. Each step should be open to scrutiny and should hold up under rigorous questioning. For example, it should be clear how respondents were identified and approached, how consent was obtained to involve respondents in the research, where and how data were collected, and how data were recorded, transcribed and stored. These are legitimate questions for the research audience and if left unanswered may raise doubts as to the quality of the research.

On the other hand, with a transparent approach to reporting the procedures for data collection, readers and recipients of the research can be confident in the quality of the research findings. The level of detail in the account of how data were accessed and handled may be limited in qualitative research, depending on the inclusion criteria of different publications and the requirements of different research audiences. However, qualitative researchers – indeed all researchers – must be able to show, upon request, how research findings were arrived at. Intellectual property rights and ethical issues of confidentiality afford protection to the researcher and respondents and are addressed later in this chapter. The important point here is to ensure that data collection techniques and approaches to data analysis are completely transparent.

Representativeness

Representativeness in qualitative research refers to the measures taken to ensure that the sample of respondents in the research study represents the population of interest to the researcher. In Chapter 2 we learnt that the number of respondents in qualitative research might be relatively small, as the aim is not to generalise to the broader population, but rather to understand from the perspective of the individual what it is like to experience a given phenomenon. In similar conditions, it may be possible to transfer the findings of a particular qualitative study to other settings. However, this is not the overall aim of qualitative research, which is to give a voice to the individual, rather than to predict for whole populations. What is important from a quality perspective is to be clear as to how the respondents in the research were identified.

A number of approaches to sampling in qualitative research are available and the researcher needs to make clear which was used. For example, qualitative researchers may take a homogeneous approach to data collection, with respondents selected in relation to specific criteria. Sample size may be limited to the availability of respondents who fit the given criteria, or by the data collection method (interviews, focus groups) or available resources. Snowball sampling is an alternative technique often used when respondents are difficult to identify. This approach allows each respondent to identify another respondent until the researcher is satisfied that the research question has been addressed or no new data is forthcoming.

An alternative method of qualitative data collection is convenience sampling, whereby the respondents are readily accessible to the researcher. Whatever the approach to data collection, the researcher must be able to justify the method in relation to issues of bias. In this sense, the latter approach is most open to question and the qualitative researcher should exhaust other forms of sampling before resorting to using convenience technique. Most importantly, the qualitative researcher should be transparent regarding the technique used and able to justify why that approach was used as opposed to an alternative. Alternative approaches should be considered and a rationale provided as to why these were not appropriate in a given research study.

The important consideration for the qualitative researcher is whether the chosen sampling technique facilitates transferability or conceptual generalisability. By this, we mean whether or not the audience can be confident that given similar situations the research findings have generated significant enough insight into the phenomenon under consideration to allow transferability to other settings.

Interpretative rigour

Interpretative rigour refers to how qualitative researchers deal with and present the data. To minimise the risk of bias within the analysis, qualitative researchers often use the notion of inter-rater reliability. Inter-rater reliability involves a process of triangulation where more than one researcher is involved in the data analysis process. In this way, the validity and reliability of qualitative data are enhanced. Transcripts are coded and themes identified by each member of the research team before being shared across the team. This process of sharing and discussion allows for a more nuanced approach to data analysis. A related technique is that of respondent validation or member checking, whereby the actual respondents in the research are given the opportunity to read and review the transcripts from their interviews. Respondent validation, if undertaken, is best performed as close in time to the actual data collection as possible, as recollection and/or interpretation of events may decrease over time.

Techniques for enhancing interpretative rigour include different methods of triangulation: for example using a variety of documentary sources, using multiple methods of data collection, or using more than one theoretical framework for data analysis.

Reflexivity

Consideration should be paid by qualitative researchers to the relationship of researcher to respondents. The nature of qualitative research in health and social care often means that the researcher is known to the respondents and familiar (if not with the respondents themselves) then with the research setting. Were this not the case, important research into aspects of health and illness would remain the remit of independent researchers with little or no insight into issues of relevance to those individuals most affected by the phenomenon under consideration, namely the patients and those involved in their care. Hence measures need to be taken by qualitative researchers to ensure that the quality of research, where researcher and respondents may be known to each other, is not compromised. Reflexivity is where open acknowledgement is made of the relationship between researcher, research topic and respondents. Qualitative researchers must be able to demonstrate how their value systems impact on the research question, design, data collection and data analysis.

Transferability

We have previously referred to transferability in qualitative research as a more appropriate concept than generalisability, given the aim of qualitative research: to understand from the individual's perspective what it is like to experience a particular phenomenon, and not to make predictions for whole populations. In terms of the quality of qualitative research, transferability or conceptual generalisability refers to how well the research findings may usefully inform healthcare settings other than the one in which the original research was undertaken. Qualitative researchers need to be mindful of claims made about their research findings and avoid overplaying or overstating the case. In order for qualitative researchers to be confident in the transferability and applicability of their research to similar healthcare settings, attention should be paid to the following:

- Clarification and justification of the research question
- Transparency in detailing the steps in the research process
- Representativeness of the sampling strategy
- Careful interpretation of the findings with useful employment of triangulation
- Consideration of the relationship between researcher, respondent and the context of the research

Ethical issues in qualitative research

Ethical approval is required for all research undertaken within the health and social care field, to protect the respondents and to ensure the maintenance of ethical standards. The National Research Ethics Service (NRES) exists to facilitate ethical research that is of potential benefit to participants, science and society, and provides an ethical review of proposed research via its Research Ethics Committees (RECs). The purpose of the REC is to ensure consideration of the rights, dignity and well-being of research participants by the researcher(s) and it is on this basis that the REC makes its decision to approve the research, to require amendments to the research proposal, or indeed to reject the proposed research. The Social Care Research Ethics Committee is part of the NRES and has a remit to review adult social care research proposals. A more thorough discussion of the role of NRES is given in Chapter 9. Universities and other organisations typically require ethical approval for research carried out by their employees, or on their behalf, including student research, and will facilitate ethical approval through their own RECs.

Research in health and social care is carried out to contribute to the health and well-being of those who take part in it. When thinking about ethical issues in research a polarisation of research into quantitative and qualitative is not helpful, as ethical issues cut across the philosophical divide. Having said that, the qualitative methods considered in this chapter, for example ethnography, phenomenology, action research and narrative methods, do pose certain ethical challenges for the researcher. We now look at these in detail.

Informed and voluntary consent

Potential participants in research must be fully informed about the nature of the research, the demands it may make on them in terms of time and resources, and the potential benefits or indeed risks associated with participation before they make a decision to take part. Informed consent not only requires that adequate information is given to participants, but also that participants are capable of comprehending the information, and have the power of free choice to participate voluntarily or to decline, without actual or perceived coercion. In this sense, informed consent is a two-step process, with information about the research provided first, usually in an information sheet, followed by written consent using a consent form.

In qualitative research data collection usually requires participants to consent to be interviewed, either face-to-face or by telephone. Interviews can be lengthy and may have the potential to cause anxiety for the respondents. It is essential that participants are aware of exactly what they are consenting to, including where the data collection process will take place, what will happen to the data once collected, how it will be stored and for how long. Participants should be informed that they have the right to withdraw from the study at any time should they wish to do so and to know what will happen to any data collected from them up to and including the point of withdrawal. Participants should be provided with details of how to complain about the conduct of the research or researchers, without having to ask for this information.

Confidentiality and anonymity of research participants

Participants in research have the right to expect that information collected from them is kept in strictest confidence. Anonymity occurs when the researcher cannot link a participant with the data collected from that participant, for example, when a questionnaire is used to collect data, and it is returned to the researcher with no identifying details on it. However, as we have seen, qualitative research involves the collection of data from individuals, in their own words, usually through interviews or focus groups. In these situations the researcher makes a promise of confidentiality to the respondent and guarantees that any information will not be publically reported or made accessible to anyone other than the research team, unless explicit consent has been obtained to do so from the participants. Consent should be obtained from participants for agreement to use direct quotations, which is often a feature of reporting qualitative data. When directly quoting respondents verbatim, i.e. word for word, the respondent is anonymised or assigned an identification number or letter. In focus groups, where a number of participants are brought together, agreement should be sought at the beginning, from all involved, to respect the right to privacy.

Doing no harm, doing good and reciprocity

In qualitative research the potential to cause physical harm to participants does not arise in the same way as it might in scientific research, for example in clinical trials of new treatments. However, it is entirely possible for psychological harm to occur during qualitative research, especially when using in-depth data collection techniques. The qualitative researcher must be mindful of this and, although not necessarily refraining from asking probing questions, must do so with sensitivity. In the event that respondents become distressed, the researcher should be prepared in advance and should have access to support for the participants and for themselves, should this become necessary.

Ethical issues in midwifery research

Midwifery practice is concerned with how midwives relate to others; how they practise midwifery; how they uphold professional responsibilities and duties; and how they are to work to assure the integrity of the profession of midwifery. Midwife researchers are, by definition, concerned with the key themes of midwifery, i.e. midwifery relationships; the practice of midwifery; professional responsibilities of midwives; and advancement of midwifery knowledge and practice. Midwifery researchers must pay particular attention to protecting the rights of the individual woman, do her no harm, obtain her informed consent, respect her individual autonomy, and act as an agent of professional, legal and moral justice (Sinclair, 2011). When carrying out research, midwife researchers must behave ethically throughout the process of conducting research in the same way that midwifery practitioners behave ethically in clinical practice. While it might be impossible when carrying out research with individual women in the real world for there to be no risk at all, nevertheless midwifery researchers must be accountable for ensuring that all steps have been taken to demonstrate good ethical practice.

Doing research and practising as a midwife at the same time can lead to ethical conflicts, as the ethical codes for midwifery practice and those for conducting research are subtly different, with the consequence that midwife-researchers may struggle with ethical considerations when doing research as a practising midwife. Key issues of concern for midwife-researchers include multiple and conflicting roles including the ethical issues of confidentiality and trust. Potential ethical dilemmas may relate to the amount of control the midwife-researcher has over the research process, especially data collection. Midwife researchers undertaking research in and on midwifery practice need to be trusted to make the best possible ethical decisions, while at the same time being fully supported to make sound ethical decisions (Ryan *et al.*, 2011).

The International Confederation of Midwives (ICM) Code of Ethics for Midwives provides guidance for good ethical practice, and can be applied equally to midwifery research. The ICM Code of Ethics for Midwives can be found at http://www.internationalmidwives.org/assets/uploads/documents/ CoreDocuments/CD2008_001%20ENG%20Code%20of%20Ethics%20 for%20Midwives.pdf

Conclusion

In conclusion, in this chapter we have looked at issues of quality in qualitative research. We focused in particular on the criteria of clarification and justi-fication, procedural rigour, representativeness, interpretation, reflexivity and evaluative rigour, and transferability, using Kitto *et al.*'s (2008) framework for addressing quality in qualitative research. We have shown that ethical issues in research are as important a consideration for the qualitative researcher as for the quantitative researcher. Ethical considerations are integral to all steps in the research process, from the initial research question through to research design, data collection and analysis, and presentation and dissemination of results. Paying attention to ethical issues in qualitative research is key to assuring the quality of the research in terms of its rigour, dependability and reliability. Researchers undertaking qualitative research in midwifery need to pay particular attention to ethical issues concerning the rights of the individual women. Good guidance is given by the International Confederation of Midwives in their Code of Ethics for Midwives.

Further reading

Bryman, A. (2001) *Quantity and Quality in Social Research*. Routledge, New York.

Flick, U. (2007) *Managing Quality in Qualitative Research*. Sage, London.

Hammersley, M. and Traianou, A. (2012) *Ethics in Qualitative Research: Controversies and Contexts*. Sage, London.

CHAPTER 5

Quantitative research: experiments

Quantitative methods are based within the scientific method. Science has a huge impact on our lives, and a vast amount of funding is poured into it all over the world. The scientific method clearly has a lot going for it, but what can it contribute to our research? Nurses and midwives have choices when it comes to using research methods. The next two chapters will explore some of the options that quantitative research can offer. It will also point out some of the limitations.

Experience of teaching quantitative research methods has shown that, on the whole, most nurses and midwives are rather reluctant to learn about this topic. If you had to, which of these blank boxes would you tick?

	Strongly disagree	Disagree	Neutral	Agree	Strongly agree
I understand a lot about quantitative research					

At the simplest level, quantitative research deals with numbers. For some people this is a real problem. However, if you are a qualified healthcare professional then by extension you must have at least a basic understanding of mathematics – which puts you in a strong position. If you can work out an intravenous drip rate or load a syringe driver with morphine, you can definitely do quantitative research. On a personal note, I only *just* passed my mathematics Scottish Ordinary Grade examination (many years ago), but I now teach quantitative data analysis to university students. Something must have changed over the years, and it is not that I became more intelligent! Other people have discovered this too. Field (2009) has produced probably the most detailed book on statistics currently available for non-statisticians and he also, in the introduction, describes how he 'turned on' to quantitative data methods late in the day, due to an excellent teacher.

Fortunately for all healthcare workers interested in quantitative methods, the days of researchers having to deal with complex formulae, usually involving Greek letters and undertaking large numbers of calculations, are now over; we have computers to do this for us. If you have the computing skills to do your monthly budget on a Microsoft Excel worksheet, you can analyse data, present your findings and publish. There are a number of computer packages available, and this book will at times refer to SPSS (formerly 'Statistical Package for the Social Sciences', now 'IBM SPSS'), which is globally one of the most widely used statistical packages.

Which statistical packages are available to you?

Here is an early exercise for you to undertake:

1. Find out which statistical package(s) are in use within your Trust or, if you are studying, within your university.
2. Find someone who can show you what it is capable of, and ask for a demonstration.
3. Think about the sort of research findings you could analyse using such a package.

A note of caution is necessary here. Although statistical packages make this analytical power available to the researcher, some of the concepts are still quite challenging. It is up to the reader to decide whether it is worth the investment. Another warning – it can be addictive!

What are the quantities in quantitative research?

Quantitative methods deal in numbers. They measure the quantity, or amount, of a phenomenon. With numbers we can give clear answers to questions, for example:

■ Does antipsychotic drug A result in better client outcomes than drug B?

- How satisfied are clients with the outreach service?
- Do students understand quantitative data analysis lectures?

This makes quantitative methods very powerful. It is easy to imagine that when considering investing millions of pounds on an intervention some hard-nosed questions will be asked. Take the first example above. Trust managers have a lot of responsibility and big budgets. Drug A is a new antipsychotic which is cheap. The board would like to use drug A for acute inpatients, but is concerned that it is not as effective as the current 'gold standard' (i.e. the best drug conventionally used), drug B. Using drug A could reduce the drug budget, but may also result in patients with uncontrolled symptoms; their recovery may take longer and there may be unpleasant side-effects resulting in longer stays over a six-monthly period – all bad outcomes for both patients and Trust. The drug may be cheaper, but not cost-effective.

If we are qualitative researchers we can investigate the *quality* of patients' experiences, and we might:

- Obtain valuable narratives regarding their stays
- Identify what was important to the clients in terms of services and care
- Possibly get a feel for how debilitating the side-effects were.

What we could not do is *quantify* it, i.e. measure *how much* better (or worse) the new drug was.

By comparison, if we are quantitative researchers, we can use established reliable and valid assessment scales and actually measure whether the clients in group A were better or worse off than those in group B *and by how much*: the differences can be quantified, or measured.

We can also pull in other data such as:

- Lengths of stay
- How many patients did not tolerate the treatment
- How many patients developed serious side-effects

We can use quantitative data analysis to present the Trust's board with a report of these findings. If you were on the board, which methods would you rely upon to make your judgement?

Main types of quantitative research

Bowling (2009) classifies quantitative research into two main groups: experimental and non-experimental. This structure will be used here. In practice, this produces two main types of exploration: the classic experiment and the survey. This is not an exhaustive classification, but it does cover the majority of the quantitative research that is published and is relevant to healthcare.

Hypotheses and research questions

The first step in designing a quantitative research project is to clarify what is to be researched. The traditional method is to set a hypothesis. A hypothesis is a statement of the researcher's expectations about the relationship between two variables. A variable is any item that can vary and be measured, for example body weight (measured in kilograms) and exercise tolerance (measured in number of metres run). Note that both of these variables can be represented mathematically.

The hypothesis is therefore a prediction that links the two, for example: 'an increase in body weight will reduce the level of exercise tolerance'. This can then be used as a basis on which to construct an experiment.

Exercise

Identify an issue within your clinical area which could be worth exploring using an experiment. Identify the two variables involved and formulate an initial hypothesis. Having done this, build in more detail. One very clear way to do this is to state who is being experimented upon. Using the example in the paragraph above, if it is formulated by a nurse working in a cardiac rehabilitation clinic, then the client group should be included:

'an increase in body weight of patients following myocardial infarction will reduce the level of exercise tolerance.'

> The more detail the better; a well-formulated hypothesis will guide the experimental design.

Null hypotheses

Traditional scientific development is built upon taking a body of knowledge, making deductions and then testing them. It is only when parts of this body of knowledge have been shown to be wrong that real scientific progress can be shown to be made. Therefore, although it seems rather complicated, in experimental research using quantitative data analysis it is more usual to form a *null hypothesis* (Parahoo, 2006), for example, 'an increase in body weight of patients following myocardial infarction will *not* reduce the level of exercise tolerance'. Null hypotheses may be scientifically desirable, but can be confusing. For this reason it is quite acceptable to stay with a standard hypothesis, particularly if it gives clear guidance as to what is being researched.

Exercise

Take your hypothesis identified above, and convert it into a null hypothesis. Does this clarify the issues for you?

Experimental research

Experimental research is derived directly from the scientific method. It is based upon two main components:

- Researchers introduce an **intervention** or **treatment**
- A measurement is made of the effect (if any) of the treatment.

If in your research question you have statements comparing one treatment with another, or exploring the effects of an intervention (e.g. education, new techniques in wound dressing or working practices), then experimental research is likely to be the way forward.

Here is an example of a very badly designed experiment that meets these criteria. Read through it and spend a few minutes answering the questions:

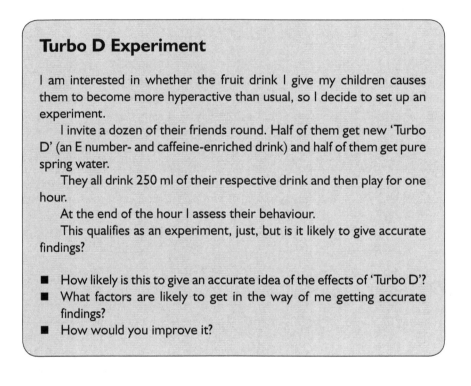

Turbo D Experiment

I am interested in whether the fruit drink I give my children causes them to become more hyperactive than usual, so I decide to set up an experiment.

I invite a dozen of their friends round. Half of them get new 'Turbo D' (an E number- and caffeine-enriched drink) and half of them get pure spring water.

They all drink 250 ml of their respective drink and then play for one hour.

At the end of the hour I assess their behaviour.

This qualifies as an experiment, just, but is it likely to give accurate findings?

- How likely is this to give an accurate idea of the effects of 'Turbo D'?
- What factors are likely to get in the way of me getting accurate findings?
- How would you improve it?

Analysis

It is possible that if carried out, this experiment might get some interesting findings, but it seems unlikely that they would be either reliable or valid. Clearly it is definitely not acceptable to carry out unannounced experiments on small children, but there are also a number of items which must be clarified.

The first one is the variables concerned. A variable is something that can be measured. Nurses and midwives are commonly involved in identifying variables in their practice:

- Dosages of drugs
- Amount of fluid input
- Amount of fluid output
- Number of weeks of gestation

Others include age, gender, shoe size etc. In quantitative research we are interested in defining the variables because this will ensure that we are very clear as to what we are measuring.

In the Turbo D experiment above, to say 'at the end of the hour I assess their behaviour' is of no value. What variables are we going to measure? Because this is quantitative research they need to be quantities which we can assign a number to. For example, I could:

- Hire a radar gun and measure the speed which the children run past me (miles per hour)
- Count the number of times they run into each other (number of collisions per minute)
- Measure the volume of noise in my garden using a sound pressure meter (decibels).

All three could be measured at the same time, perhaps to pick up on different aspects of their behaviour. Therefore if the variables can be defined, we can start to be clear as to exactly what we are measuring, and hence the effect of the drink.

The next item is the *sample* of children. Twelve is a very small number to include in any experiment and causes a problem. I may already have a number of hyperactive children in the group, because one of my children is himself hyperactive. Whatever happens to the group, it is likely that these children will produce atypical findings, they will introduce *bias*. This means that the group will not behave as a more representative group of 'normal' children would.

Finally, consent is a major issue. Clearly it is not acceptable to experiment in a haphazard way with children, who constitute a vulnerable group. In experiments in healthcare, people themselves are experimented upon, their treatments are changed and they may be exposed to hazard. Experimental research therefore requires stringent ethical consideration. For those interested, a useful starting point is the National Research Ethics Service (NRES) homepage (NRES, 2013).

The Turbo D experiment, for all its faults, does however contain the basic structure of an experiment.

Constructing an experiment: some terminology

Quantitative research has its own terminology and it is worth becoming familiar with it. The special characteristic of an experiment which sets it apart from all other types of design is the ability to show *cause* and *effect*. This means that if you wish to introduce a new treatment, then setting up an experiment will give you the evidence to show that the treatment either works or does not work, meaning that if the treatment is introduced (cause) it will have a predictable outcome (effect) on a *population*.

The population is the group of people whose behaviour you wish to be able to explore or predict. In the Turbo D example, the group might be children between the ages of 10 and 12 living in England. Clearly it would be impossible to experiment with this whole population, so a *sample* is chosen, the maximum size commonly being limited by the resources available to the researcher. If the sample is chosen carefully then it should be possible to transfer or generalise the findings to the larger population.

The treatment which is manipulated is termed the *independent variable* e.g. the administration of Turbo D in the previous example. This compared with a control treatment. In the healthcare setting this is usually described as a 'gold standard' conventional treatment. This means that if the patient is not included in the experimental group, they can be assured that they will get the best conventional treatment, as decided by existing evidence.

The *dependent variable* is what you measure. In the Turbo D example this was not specified, but some options have been outlined above. One or more of these variables could be chosen. Figure 5.1 (see p. 75) shows the main items within an experiment, including the particulars of the 'Turbo D' design.

Here is an example from healthcare science. Thomas *et al.* (2009) set up an experiment to compare two non-pharmacological methods for treating clients with asthma in primary care. One hundred and eighty three asthma clients were randomised into two groups. This means that each client had the same chance of being in one or the other group. This again reduces the likelihood of bias. The comparison was between two groups: those who received physiotherapist-supervised breathing training (the independent variable) and nurse delivered asthma education (the control group). The dependent variables were numerous, but one of the main items was the Asthma Quality of Life Questionnaire (AQLQ), which has been shown in other studies to be sensitive to the well-being of asthma patients. The experiment showed that at one month there were similar scores between the two groups, but at six months the breathing training resulted in more favourable scores. This experiment shows a clear cause and effect, and it can be concluded that if breathing specialists are in a position to provide one of the two treatments, there is a strong case to use breathing training.

Controlling the experiment

As shown in this example, in a healthcare setting, the independent and control variables can be complex. Imagine you are a patient undergoing major surgery and are approached by a researcher exploring pain control. You might, initially at least, be interested in helping with their research. Most patients are well disposed to help promote care. However, if the choice was that one half of the patients received a new promising drug for pain control (independent variable), or to have a placebo – i.e. no effective pain relief (control variable), then only the very brave or very foolish would take part.

In healthcare, then, the most common contrast is between the experimental treatment (dependent variable), and what can be described as a 'Gold Standard Conventional Treatment' (control variable). This is also a part of the ethical process. NHS Trust Ethical Committees, NRES and practitioners themselves have a duty to safeguard the participants of experiments. They insist, therefore, that at worst the participants will have a good standard of treatment, one that is research- and evidence-based, and is thoroughly up to date. This will then be compared with the experimental treatment, which has been shown in preliminary trials (also termed Phase I and II trials; to be discussed later), to be likely to be at least as good as, and possibly better than, the Gold Standard.

Therefore, taking the example of the surgical patient already mentioned, the independent variable is the new drug and it would be compared with an agreed standard intervention which has been shown to deliver good quality pain relief – a patient-controlled opioid system, for example.

Dependent variable

This is what is measured. The experiment is designed so that changes due to the manipulation of independent variables are picked up by the dependent variable, either immediately or later. For example, changes in pain using the surgical experiment outlined above could be assessed in a number of ways:

- Patients are asked to use a visual analogue scale every hour where they score their pain on a scale from 0–10.
- Heart rate and blood pressure are recorded (the basis here is physiological, that pain would cause an increase in both).
- Patients are given a questionnaire on discharge, asking them how well they felt their pain was controlled.

Clearly, a lot of expertise is required to pick sensitive and relevant dependant variables, and this is at the heart of good experimental design. To help with this it is worth taking time and scholarship to develop a detailed research question or hypothesis.

Randomising the experiment

The primary reason for random assignment is to remove the potential of bias in the assignment of people to one intervention or another. Kunz *et al.* (2007) conducted a Cochrane Review comparing randomised and non-randomised trials and found that the latter tended to produce a larger effect size by on average 25%, suggesting that non-randomisation included positive bias within the design, although they also found that it was important to conceal allocation (or in the jargon, to 'blind' – see also under the Hawthorne Effect). Randomisation is in principle simple. For example in a simple experimental design with two groups, for each participant a coin is tossed. If it lands heads up, the participant is allocated to the control group, if it lands tails up, the participant is allocated to the experimental group. We can do this with confidence, because we know that if a coin is tossed and caught, as long as the sample is large enough (e.g. 100 tosses), then approximately half the time it will land heads up and half face up. This is fine, if rather laborious, but of course does not work if more than two options are available. If there are three or more, another option is required. Polit and Beck (2008) describe the use of a set of random numbers, which is very clear. Rather than repeat this, we will discuss another method.

Randomisation exercise

Enter *'random number generator'* into your computer's search engine. You will find many free examples. A very simple one to use is provided by Random. Org (http://www.random.org/). To generate a random allocation, you need to input the number of choices (the default is 100). For this example, we shall assume that your experimental design has three groups (Control, Group A, Group B). Then the maximum (max) will be a value of three as shown:

True Random Number Generator

Min: 1

Max: 3

Generate

Result:

Powered by RANDOM.ORG

Each time you click *Generate*, a random number between 1 and 3 inclusive is generated. Here is a stream of digits generated by repeating this 42 times (to allow the possibility of perfect allocation, a multiple of three was chosen):

```
1  2  2  1  3  1  3  2  3  1  2  3  2  3
2  3  1  1  3  1  2  3  2  3  3  3  2  1
1  2  3  1  3  1  1  2  3  2  1  3  2  2
```

As this is quite a small sample size, although the groups are completely random (there is no pattern to allocation), they are slightly uneven (13 ones, 14 twos and 15 threes). Inconsistencies such as these will even out as the sample gets larger.

Beware of casual use of the term *randomisation*. For example, if exploring pain in patients following orthopaedic surgery, the following ways of randomising the sample are all comprehensively *wrong*:

1. Patients on a Tuesday are allocated to the control; patients on a Wednesday are allocated to the treatment.
2. Patients having surgery in the morning are allocated to the control, patients having surgery in the afternoon are allocated to the treatment.
3. Patients are allocated according to their surname: all those whose surnames are within the first 13 letters (A–M) are allocated to the control, all those within the last 13 are allocated to the treatment.

These are not examples of randomisation because (among other possibilities):

1. Different surgeons typically operate on different days. One may typically have more major cases than his or her colleague, such that the Tuesday cases have more pain than the Wednesday ones. This would then bias the results.
2. The surgical teams (and nurses) may all be fresh and raring to go at 09:00 in the morning. Come 13:00, they may start to feel fatigue, or have a post-prandial dip, such that their work and pain relief is less than perfect, which could all bias the results.
3. Different surnames may represent different ethnicities. For example, it has been noted that a lot of African surnames begin with the letter M. Whether people of African extraction are particularly stoic, or sensitive to pain, or just the same as everyone else, is outside the scope of this discussion, but nonetheless, this example shows how using this criterion could again introduce bias.

This brief discussion gives examples of how inadvertent variables can result in a move away from true research findings and result in the possible introduction of bias. These inadvertent factors are described as *confounding variables*, and a lot of research design is really about trying to rule out as many confounding variables as possible. This will be illustrated in the next exercise.

Sampling in experimental research

The basic principles of sampling in experimental research are quite straight-forward. The researcher wishes to measure the impact of the treatment within a population. If resources such as time, money and administrative staff were available, the entire population would be included in the research. This is seldom possible, so a smaller representative sample is selected. Whenever a sample is chosen, there is the opportunity to introduce sampling error, which can produce *bias* (Sapsford, 2007). Bias means a deviation from the true value of the population, and is due to a wide range of variability within people.

Exercise

Figure 5.1 shows the basic structure of an experiment which has been annotated to show the variables in the Turbo D example. Using the hypothesis you produced earlier in the chapter, take five minutes to draw your own version. Identify and include the independent and dependent variables. Give as much detail as you can, including for example, the length of time between manipulating the independent variable and measuring the dependent one. Try to reduce the number of confounding variables as much as possible.

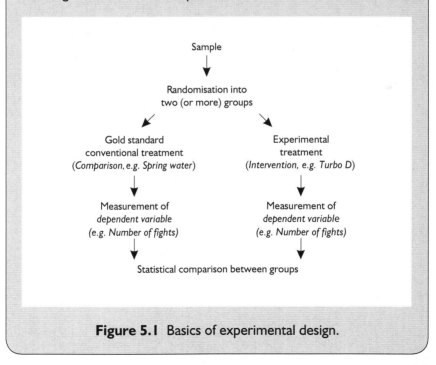

Figure 5.1 Basics of experimental design.

By definition, not everyone can be included within a sample. Results in this situation are likely to be skewed, i.e. pushed away from more representative values. As anyone who has worked in healthcare knows, people come in a wide variety of sizes, shapes and responses to even the most straightforward suggestions. If a sample of 10 subjects is used within a research project, it can be conjectured that one or two extreme cases will produce unrepresentative or biased results. If the sample is then increased to 100 or 1,000 subjects, the unrepresentative subjects are likely to become progressively diluted. Therefore in quantitative research, in general, the larger the sample size, the better (Shields and Twycross, 2008).

How large should a sample be?

Power analysis is the branch of statistics which shows the size of sample that is required to distinguish an effect in, for example, an experimental setting. It is not intended in this book to explore power analysis in great detail, but there are some basic rules:

- The larger the difference in the dependent variable between groups (*effect size*), the easier it is to detect; therefore fewer participants are required in the design.
- Some statistical techniques are more able to distinguish differences between groups (they are described as being *more powerful*) than others.
- Design and sample size depend on how much the researcher wishes to expose themselves to error; if they are very cautious, then again a larger size is required.

There are two types of error. Type 1 error is where it appears that there is a difference between groups, but in fact *it is not real* (or statistically significant). This is also known as false positive error. Type 2 error is where it appears as though there is no difference between two groups, but in fact *there really is*. This is also known as false negative error (Greasley, 2008). The power of the design is calculated by subtracting the Type 2 error value from 1. As can be seen, this is quite complex and whole books have been written about power analysis. For a good summary which is easy to read, try page 12 of Anthony (1999).

Another way to avoid too much theory is to use a statistical package to predict sample size. One excellent example of this is G*Power, which also has the advantage of being free. It originates in the Heinrich Heine University in Dusseldorf. At the time of writing (early 2013) it can be downloaded from http://www.psycho.uni-duesseldorf.de/abteilungen/aap/gpower3/.

Sample size: some rules of thumb

Running some examples using G*Power allows us to make some broad predictions, which might be useful if the student wishes to make a research proposal. These examples are based upon using a *t*-test to detect differences between two groups. This is one of the standard tests used within experiments and is quite powerful. G*Power uses Cohen's widely used criteria for weak, medium and strong effects, and for the technically minded, Type 1 error was set at 0.05 and power at 0.8 (these are standard criteria as outlined in Anthony, 1999):

- If an experiment has 50 participants, split into two groups, it is only likely to be able to detect a large difference between groups.
- If an experiment has 130 participants, split into two groups, it is likely to be able to detect a medium or large strength difference between groups.
- If an experiment has 800 participants, split into two groups, it is likely to be able to detect a weak, medium or large strength difference between groups.

From this discussion it can be seen that if we are interested in effects which have real clinical significance, i.e. are at least of medium effect, then a sample size of greater than 130 will be required to produce findings which may have impact in the real word, i.e. identify at least medium effects. To summarise, the message is quite clear: in quantitative research a large sample size will support the ability to pick up differences between groups, and the larger the better!

Calculating effect size

Here is an example of one calculation to determine effect size, Cohen's *d*. This is named after Jacob Cohen (1923–1998), who wrote a very influential book that really forms the basis of much modern-day power analysis (Cohen, 1988). This is used in studies that have two groups and are normally distributed. If you are not familiar with the terms 'mean' and 'standard deviation', you may prefer to wait until you have read the worked examples in Chapter 7, and then return to this calculation.

The heart rate of two groups of students was measured. Group A had an average rate of 80.75 bpm, Group B of 84.05 bpm. The standard deviation for Group A was 8.48, and for Group B 7.05.

To work out the effect size, the two mean values are subtracted from each other, and this value is then divided by the mean standard deviation. Note that whether the effect size is negative or positive does not matter; therefore this will be ignored:

$$\text{Effect size} = \frac{(\text{Mean Group A} - \text{Mean Group B})}{(\text{SD Group A} + \text{SD Group B}) \times 0.5}$$

$$= \frac{(80.75 - 84.04)}{(8.48 + 7.05) \times 0.5}$$

$$= \frac{-3.29}{7.76}$$

$$= -0.42$$

Cohen gives three broad ranges for effect size:

Small	0.20–0.49
Medium	0.50–0.70
Large	0.80+

Therefore our calculated effect size is essentially quite small (the negative sign can be ignored – it is the size of the difference which is of interest), and therefore we would need quite a large sample size in an experimental design. If we then want to know how large, then again we would use G*Power. Using the previous settings (two-tailed test, alpha = 0.05, power = 0.8) plus the *d* calculated (0.42), the programme tells us that we would need a total sample size of 142.

If we do not have a sample as large as this, then there is another option. G*Power allows us to plot effect size against total sample size:

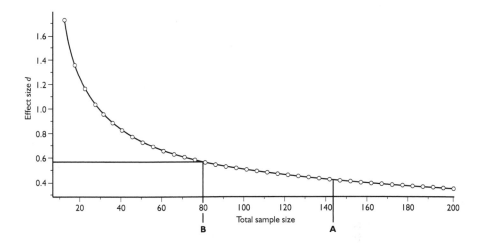

The line labelled 'A' reflects the above power calculation. If you then travel horizontally from where the sample size of 142 touches the curved line, this takes you to the calculated effect size of 0.42. However, if we only have 80 participants, (as shown by line 'B'), then we can expect to pick up effects sized 0.58 and above, e.g. using Cohen's criteria 'medium'. This may be perfectly acceptable, but would be identified as a limitation when writing up the study.

Sampling strategies

There is more to sampling in quantitative research than just getting the largest feasible number of subjects, however. It is important to have a clear sampling strategy, so that the group identified in the research hypothesis is represented fully in the research itself, otherwise the research will not be valid.

Probability sampling

In probability sampling, a formal attempt is made to represent the population within the sample. It can also be described as a strategy in which each member of the population has an equal chance of being selected. There are many sampling strategies in print, and often different terms are used to describe similar strategies. What follows is a reasonably simple category of sampling strategies which, from reading healthcare research, describes perhaps 95% of the published literature. It is based upon principles found in Bowling (2009) and Polit and Beck (2008).

Random sampling

This is the most straightforward and rigorous way to undertake probability sampling. A random sample is taken from the population up to a predetermined maximum number. Random means to have no specific pattern, purpose or objective. In more scientific terms, and applied to sampling, it means that each person within the group has the same likelihood of being chosen. This means that subjects or events are chosen with no pattern at all between them. The classic example of this is to make a list of names of subjects, cut the list up, fold them over and put them in a hat (or other receptacle). The names are then taken out one by one until the sample is complete. Each name has the same chance as any other to be included within the sample. This is such a powerful technique that it has actually escaped from research terminology and become part of everyday English, we may talk about 'taking a name out of the hat' to suggest some sort of sampling in common situations. This works well for small projects, but more sophisticated methods have been developed using computer-generated randomised tables.

Randomisation is the classic 'scientific' sampling method, but it relies on large samples to represent the population. It has already been suggested that within an experiment, subjects are randomised into two (or more) treatment groups. This is seen as being of great significance in the evidence-based practice movement, supporters of which would argue that without true randomised sampling, it is impossible for an experiment to illustrate cause and effect.

Stratified sampling

A stratified sample is one which the individual has an equal chance of being chosen in relation to their proportion of membership of a group within the total population. This is particularly valuable within the healthcare setting, where different groups of individuals have different needs and expectations. Healthcare practitioners in the UK, for example, are currently differentiated in work and payment by their pay bands. When undertaking research with a group of workers, it might be felt necessary to include a proportion from each band to get the full picture of the workforce. This is particularly useful in survey research. Strictly, there should be a proportionate selection from each group (stratum means a layer; hence stratified) as shown in Table 5.1.

Table 5.1

Agenda for Change banding	5	6	7
Total number of staff	300	100	50
Number include in sample	60	20	10

In this example, a 20% sample has been taken from each pay band within the population, so that the researcher can be confident that the proportion of subjects from each pay band is the same in the sample as it is in the wider population. Sampling can then take place within the strata, ideally using randomisation. One point to note here is that if the sample was large enough, all groups would be proportionately presented. Stratified sampling is therefore very useful in the situation where a smaller sample only can be used.

Inclusive sampling

An inclusive sample is one in which everyone within the population is included. This is in many ways the ideal, as it removes the possibility of bias within the sample, by definition. However, it depends on the size of a population as to whether this is possible. It is a very attractive sampling strategy within some healthcare settings, when relatively small populations are sampled. For example, if undertaking research regarding hand washing by midwives within a hospital ward, there might only be 30–40 individuals to sample from. The simplest strategy is then to include the whole population within the research. The limiting factor becomes the researcher's resources and ability to deal with the full population. Nursing and midwifery research is often placed within a ward or community setting. In this type of setting inclusive sampling may be easily achieved. Note that if an inclusive sample is used, then bias is avoided by definition; the sample *is* the population.

Non-probability sampling

It may not be possible to gain access to the full population. If this is the case, then a non-probability sampling technique may be necessary. This means that there is no sustained effort to represent the entire population. Instead, the researcher effectively samples as many subjects as he or she can, using the resources available to them. These techniques largely *do not* use a random sample and some bias will probably be involved. Therefore if used with an experimental design, these techniques introduce limitations which should be addressed within the research team, and discussed when writing the experiment up. If resources are limited (which is usually the case), although less than ideal, these techniques may still allow robust research to take place.

Purposive sampling

This is a branch of non-probability sampling. The researcher identifies the quality which makes the sample group relevant to the researcher. For example, an educationalist might wish to sample students from Years 1, 2 and 3 of a midwifery programme. A sample of the students is then accessed and invited to take part. It is the 'hand picked' nature of the subjects that distinguishes purposive (sometimes called purposeful) sampling; it means that although the subjects will all be directly relevant to the research (an advantage), the sample is specialised and probably biased and may not be applicable to the wider population (a disadvantage). Again, for experimental research this means that the ability to justify cause and effect becomes limited, but it does not mean that the research becomes invalid. It means rather that the findings have to be applied with care and the limitation of the sampling should be acknowledged.

Convenience sampling

This is the weakest form of sampling to be discussed here. Literally it means that the selection of subjects suits the convenience of the researcher: e.g. the researcher chooses the first five subjects to come through the door, or similar method of access. Typically this is as a result of having limited resources, but as discussed above, although it is a limitation to the quality of the research, it does not make good-quality research impossible. It does, however, move further way from linking cause to effect and produces yet more caution in applying findings to practice. Using the example of the students above, if the first 50 students to enter the coffee room on campus are chosen, the sample is likely to be biased – they may make an unrepresentative proportion of caffeine-depleted, and hence possibly depressed, subjects, and quite possibly should be avoided.

Similarly, within practice, if the first five patients on a morning list for minor surgery are sampled there is likely to be bias; the consultant may have arranged for the more straightforward cases to be dealt with first.

Randomised Controlled Trials (RCTs)

In some ways RCTs represent the most formal scientific approach to research. RCTs are very highly specified experiments. They are important because if a company wishes to launch a new drug or medical procedure onto the market, there are very high standards to be met to ensure that it is (a) safe, (b) likely to be better than currently existing drugs and (c) cost-effective. To do this, RCTs are used in healthcare, education and other fields. These provide evidence to statutory bodies. In the UK, for example, if there is any concern that a treatment may not be effective or will be prohibitively expensive, the National Institute for Health and Clinical Excellence (NICE) will investigate to confirm that the treatments represent best practice and best care. A similar role is undertaken in the USA by the United States Food and Drug Administration.

There are classically four phases in an RCT (adapted from Polit and Beck, 2008):

■ **Phase I: Safety, feasibility, acceptability**
The inventors of the new treatment feel that they have a promising product and start to explore its properties. Moving from animal trials to humans, they explore useful doses, safety and possible side-effects. At the end of the Phase I trials, the researchers will have an idea of whether the drug is likely to harm anyone, and how to use it. Typically this takes place outside of the NHS and is run by private companies and clinics.

■ **Phase II: Preliminary effect size, side effects, dosing**

Evidence is built up exploring the effectiveness of the treatment. Phase II uses small trials and commonly some quasi-experimental designs to build up a picture of the possible clinical use of the product. This phase can be described as a pilot or exploratory stage.

■ **Phase III: Efficacy of new treatment compared to standard**

This is the full experimental test of the treatment. Typically it takes place (in UK healthcare) within NHS settings. It is a full experiment, and contains a number of elements. As a piece of high-quality experimental research, a large sample size is necessary. This may include hundreds or even thousands of subjects. The control group is supplied by using a 'Gold Standard' conventional treatment. This must be based upon the latest available evidence in order to gain ethical approval for the trial. As the name suggests, randomisation of the sample is important. The split between the control and experimental group is provided by a randomised process, so that participants have an equal chance of being in either group. To obtain a large sample size, RCTs are commonly spread over a number of sites, and may be termed 'multi-centre'. To minimise the introduction of bias, groups are commonly 'blinded', an unfortunate term which means that they are unaware of which treatment is being used. With

The Hawthorne Effect

Blinding is designed to minimise the 'Hawthorne Effect'. The Hawthorne Works was a factory near Chicago USA which produced all the switches for American telephones – it was a big factory. In the mid-1920s its working practices were explored by researchers. It was found that whenever the researchers were present, productivity increased. In research terms, an unacknowledged independent variable was the knowledge that the workers were being studied. Similar effects can be suggested that are relevant to healthcare. For example, if it is known that staff are being observed as they wash their hands, then it is likely that, during the study, staff will take more time to wash their hands, and be more particular as they do it. Once the study is over, staff become more relaxed and will probably move back to their previous habits.

single blinding, the subject is not aware of whether they are in the experimental or control group. With double blinding, neither patient nor clinical staff are aware of which treatment is in place.

■ **Phase IV: Application in clinical setting long-term safety**
Once the treatment has been adopted and is in practice, this is not the end of the story. The long-term effectiveness of the medication is researched plus the occurrence of side-effects. In time, new interventions and drugs will be produced, and further comparisons will be made, through experimental and other forms of research.

Impact of RCTs

RCTs contribute directly to clinical decision making. They are described as being high-quality evidence (Grey, 2009). Here is an example. There is a condition called essential thrombocythaemia in which the bone marrow produces too many platelets. As a result, people with this condition are at risk of thromboses and, if the count is very high, of bleeding. An RCT was undertaken, called the PT-1 Trial, taking subjects from New Zealand, the UK, Australia and France. It compared two drug treatments: hydroxycarbamide plus low-dose aspirin and anagrelide plus low-dose aspirin. So strong were the findings that hydroxycarbamide plus aspirin was the better treatment (at least for high-risk patients) that the trial was halted, and this is the recommendation used widely in the UK (Harrison *et al.*, 2005). This information has been made widely available to the public through educational materials, such as those produced by Leukaemia Research (Campbell, 2006).

More complex designs

The RCTs we have looked at have all used simple random allocation into two groups. More complex designs, however, may be required. Two straightforward variations are where (1) the independent variable, for example a drug, is given in two different dosages, therefore requiring three randomised groups: Control, Dosage 1 and Dosage 2, and (2) where there is more than one independent variable included, for example Drug A and Drug B versus Control. Again three randomised groups would be required: Control, Drug A and Drug

B. More groups can of course be included, but at this point the total number of people who would need to be recruited in order that the experiment have sufficient power starts to get larger (see also the section on power analysis). This is not necessarily a problem if you are fortunate enough to have a sufficiently large budget.

The RCTs that have been discussed so far can all be described as post-test only designs. This means that the measurement of the dependent variable is made only at the end of the experiment. This is the simplest design, but others may be useful.

Pre-test–post-test designs

In a pre-test–post-test design, a comparison is made between the participants before the intervention (the pre-test measurement) and afterwards (the post-test measurement). This works well for measuring changes in a group, particularly when they are non-homogeneous, e.g. there are quite large variations between individuals. This is actually a family of designs, and another example is given when quasi-experimental designs are discussed. Figure 5.2 shows one that involves randomisation and a control, and therefore qualifies as a true experiment:

The participants are randomised into two groups. The pre-test measurement is taken before the intervention and so provides a baseline, so that the post-test measurement allows a precise measurement of change during the experiment. An example of this is the study by Hersey *et al.* (2012). This group conducted a pre-test–post-test RCT measuring the effect of a community weight management intervention. A group of overweight participants were randomised to one of three interventions to explore if they had an effect on weight loss. The three variables were: written materials and Internet access (Group 1); the above, *plus* an interactive Internet site (Group 2); all of the above *plus* brief telephone or email coaching (Group 3). Measurements of a range of dependent variables were made at four times: baseline, 6, 12 and 15–18 months. The dependent variables measured included weight loss, physical activity and blood pressure.

Use a flow chart diagram as in Figure 5.2, to summarise the experimental design used by Hersey *et al.* (2012).

In practice, a pre-test–post-test design using randomisation is quite a rare design, but most RCTs will include a pre-intervention measurement, taken either before or after randomisation. This allows the researchers to assess how effective the randomisation was – if there are statistically significant differences between the two groups before the intervention, then there is clearly a problem with the research process; perhaps another method of randomisation is required, or a larger sample may be required to even out the differences between groups.

Crossover trials

This is the final trial type to be discussed here, although there are many more variants possible. In the simplest form of crossover trial, participants are randomised to one of two groups. One group receives treatment A (the control, for example) whilst the second group receives treatment B (the new medication). After the effects of these have been found by measurement of a suitable dependent variable, the crossover takes place, so that the first group then receives treatment B and the second group receives treatment A (Figure 5.3). Again, the dependent variable is measured.

Note that this design has balance, in that all participants are exposed to treatments A and B, although not necessarily in that order. The main benefit

Figure 5.2

for a crossover design is that each individual serves as his or her own control, which allows the design to be statistically powerful – a smaller sample size may be required than in a non-crossover design.

However, the crossover is a complex design. In addition to the basic requirements, a period of 'washout' is usually built in, so that any effect caused by the first treatment is no longer present when the next treatment commences. This means they require a longer period than other designs, and because of this, participants over a period of time may become lost to the study. This could be for a number of reasons: they may move, or their diagnosis may change, or they may even die. All of these can lead to loss of sample size and possible unbalancing of the design. For this same reason, they are of little use for a condition which is short term – it may be physically impossible to assign to the two groups if the condition has resolved within the time limit of the study (Sibbald, 1998). This can cause real problems: Frei *et al.* (2007), in a randomised crossover trial of homeopathic treatments for hyperactivity, found that they could not control for a strong carryover effect diminishing the apparent difference between placebo and treatment, despite a 12 month washout phase.

Should I take part in RCTs?

This is inevitably a personal choice. Occasionally subjects taking part in trials are featured in the news. For example in 2006 a Phase I trial of an anti-inflammatory drug TGN1412 was started in the UK. This left six volunteers seriously ill and two, at one point, possibly close to death. Fortunately, all eventually survived. However, by their nature Phase I and II trials have an element of

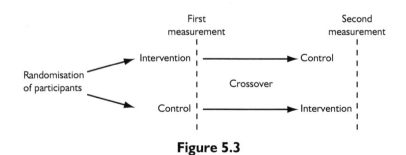

Figure 5.3

risk, and this is why subjects are paid to take part – in the case of TGN1412, it was reported that volunteers were paid £2,000 each (Rosenbaum, 2006).

There is a much stronger case to be made for taking part in Phase III trials. By this stage, manufacturers will already have a good understanding of the drug (for example). More significantly, they will have managed to convince a formal ethical committee that their drug is likely to be at least as good as conventional treatments, and there is likelihood that it may actually be better. So, if taking part and receiving the test drug, a positive case can be made for a good outcome. However, this is also the case if given the control, because part of the research design is an assurance that all non-experimental group subjects will be given up-to-date evidence-based treatment. Therefore, if given an opportunity to take part in a Phase III trial, there is some evidence that it is likely to be of benefit to the subject in either arm of the trial. This is one case of philanthropy also being of self-benefit.

Quasi-experimental designs

By now you should be able to identify each element in an RCT. All RCTs are true experiments. If any of these elements are absent, then the design may be referred to as a quasi-experimental design, i.e. they are almost, but not quite, true experiments (*quasi* literally means 'half'). The most common type is where randomisation is missing; this means that control of allocation to group will be imperfect. Quasi-experimental designs are actually a family of designs. Here are two hypothetical designs (Figures 5.4 and 5.5) and explanations of why these designs might be suitable.

In Figure 5.4, two delivery wards A and B were chosen to take part in a (quasi-) experiment. Ward B was given a new electronic system for maintaining patient records, where the clinical area became essentially paperless and all documentation was electronically recorded. The hypothesis is that if patient records were handled in this (hopefully) efficient manner, then more time would be liberated for patient care. Therefore the amount of time spent with patients might be a suitable measure.

However, the working practices in the two wards might be slightly, or even greatly different, so to control for this a pre-test–post-test design could be chosen, which could control for a number of variables – the differences between the two measures might then be more reasonably explained by the intervention. Therefore a baseline measurement could be taken and the independent variable (the new computerised system) implemented. After a suitable period of time, perhaps six months, the post-test measurement would be taken, again measuring the amount of time the midwives spent with their patients. Statistical analysis would then identify whether there was a statistically significant difference between the two, and this would show whether the system really did liberate time for hands-on caring.

Because this is a quasi-experimental study, without randomisation, this does not necessarily show true cause and effect. However, in this case, randomisation may not be possible. The systems require extensive investment, hardware, wiring up and training for the staff. Staff could not be randomised to one ward or the other on a day-to-day basis. Therefore although this quasi-experimental pre- and post-test design is not as strong a source of evidence as a true RCT, it may be the best design available within a set budget or resources.

Figure 5.5 stays with the paperless ward example, as above. In this case, the design is actually simpler. Ward A is the only participating venue and there is no comparator; instead, the electronic system is implemented after the baseline measurement. Effectively, Ward A is its own control. It can be argued that this design is weaker because it is at risk of more uncontrolled variables. For example, if there were a major round of job cuts during the implementation of the system, this would be completely uncontrolled for; was less time spent

Figure 5.4 Quasi-experimental design 1.

Figure 5.5 Quasi-experimental design 2.

with patients because of the new system or because there were fewer mid-wives to care for the patients in total?

Summary

Experiments remain a mainstay of scientific enquiry. If correctly set up and conducted they can identify cause and effect, which no other form of research can. Their scientific pedigree is both their strength and weakness. They can show the connection between variables, but because of this they may have limited use for both midwives and nurses. Both these professions, by definition, deal with delivering care to clients. Clients are almost infinitely complex and may be better served by non-deductive methods, such as qualitative research, to investigate their worlds. Similarly, it may not be possible to construct experiments on complex issues which involve degrees of patient choice. If this is the case, a survey is one form of quantitative research that can be more flexible in investigation.

CHAPTER 6

Quantitative research: surveys

Surveys are possibly the most commonly undertaken form of research. They are so popular that they have 'escaped' into everyday usage. Most readers will at some time have completed a survey, perhaps in the high street, or by post from their bank (for example), to provide market information.

Surveys are rightly popular because they are extremely flexible and can be constructed and modified to answer a wide variety of research questions. They are very good at showing *association*, but not causality. For example, a survey could be undertaken of nursing students asking them about their use of cannabis and their mood state. There is a lot of interest currently in this topic, and it has been suggested that forms of high-strength cannabis, such as 'skunk', may precipitate mental health changes. It might be found that students who smoke cannabis indeed have a lower mood state than those who do not, but this does not prove that the cannabis caused this. It might instead be hypothesised that students with a low mood state are likely to seek out cannabis for relief. The association between the two may be shown, but not proof that one causes the other. If cause and effect is required, then an experimental structure is required. This, however, is probably impossible. No ethical committee would agree to a research project where large groups of nursing students were given cannabis and were told to smoke it!

In this sort of situation, a survey may be the only suitable research design that is available. This gets close to the difference between surveys and experiments. In a survey, there is no manipulation of variables, while in experiments there is. In more common language, in a survey, a snapshot, or series of snapshots, is taken of the population. In an experiment, some aspect of the way people are treated is changed, and the effect of this is measured.

There is some common ground. Within an experiment a survey-style questionnaire may be included (commonly referred to as a data collection tool) to measure the dependent variable. Surveys should not be seen as a poor relation to experimental work: they can provide valuable information and, if well constructed, may answer the research question in good detail.

Research questions in healthcare

As has been discussed, healthcare research embraces both quantitative and qualitative methods. The use of a hypothesis, null or otherwise, is necessary for the traditional scientific way of exploring issues, and so works well for experiments. In non-experimental research it is more common to use a research question. There are a number of reasons for this. Certainly in inductive, qualitative work we cannot really identify the variables we will be working with; instead, the work is commonly designed to find what the variables are, rather than to test them. The enquiry is therefore more tentative, or open-ended; there is no pre-existing model to predict which variables will affect the results. One way to address this is to use a looser structure to start the enquiry, and this is often posed as a research question (Polit and Beck, 2008).

When deriving a research question, it is still possible to include variables that have been identified as being worthy of exploration. Here is a hypothesis used in the previous chapter:

'Increase in body weight will reduce the level of exercise tolerance.'

By comparison a more open-ended *research question* could be:

'How does increase in body weight affect the way people exercise?'

When phrased this way, the question is more open and less predictive. This allows a more creative process of research. The answer is not going to be *yes* or *no*.

Using research questions in higher degrees

This approach can be particularly useful if you want to include qualitative elements of study – a common strategy with higher degrees. For example, PhD studies collect findings over a period of three years (full-time) or five years (part-time). Within this time frame they may have two, three or even more phases of their project (Holloway and Walker, 2000; Phillips and Pugh, 2005).

Commonly, the first step of the research is to find out which variables are the important ones in a particular setting.

Here is an example from a real-life PhD, exploring how the use of a computerised data management system would affect nurses working within critical care. To start with, even if pressed to do so, it would have been impossible to state a hypothesis, because it was not clear what the variables were. Instead, to guide the study an open-ended research question was posed ('What are the factors that affect the way nurses use a computerised data management system?'), and this gave guidance to the first qualitative phase, which used interviews to identify the main issues. It was then possible to set up a compara-

---

Exercise: setting a research question

A clear and simple research question is a good start to a research project using a survey.

Most research questions have two main items:

- Who is going to be researched?
- What is the focus of the research?

Take a look around your clinical area and identify an aspect of practice that you think could be improved. Draft your research question as one simple question, for example:

'How do midwives promote breast feeding in mothers during the first 24 hours following delivery?'

In this case it is clear who is being researched: it is the midwives working in delivery wards. There is also clarity regarding the focus of the work, including specific details of the group of women they care for. This is quite different from formulating a hypothesis. It is more open-ended, it predicts less and it gives freedom to choose a range of research tactics. This question could be explored using a survey.

Look at the research question you have drafted; is it clear who will be researched and is it clear what the main focus will be? If you are looking for the relationship between two variables, then an experiment may be the best way to proceed; if the question is open-ended, then a survey may be the best way to proceed.

tive quantitative exploration to identify which of these variables were important, in a similar way to setting up an experiment.

In summary, therefore, the use of a research question works well for mixed method designs, where a hypothesis would be too limiting. It also works well for surveys.

What is a survey?

Surveys have a long history. Sapsford (2007) identifies that the 11th century Domesday Book is one of the earliest surveys, listing all the manors and farms of England for the purpose of taxation. This meaning of surveying survives as a term used in geography and architecture; before buying a house, we have it surveyed to find its value and identify any architectural problems.

The sort of survey to be discussed here is more specialised. Although qualitative surveys are feasible, this chapter will focus on the more common quantitative research surveys, using systematic methods to gather specific information from a specific population. To do this, it is wise to start with a clear research question, which can be used to construct a suitable questionnaire that will produce reliable and valid findings (Bowling and Ibrahim, 2005).

Types of survey

With a *direct survey*, the researcher typically approaches a sample of the target group and may interview them or ask them to fill in a questionnaire.

With an *indirect survey*, written oral and visual records can be surveyed; a popular option here might be to explore patient/client records. Data will usually be entered in a data collection tool, so again production of a clear, structured questionnaire is at the centre of a well-conducted survey. There are a number of ways to conduct a survey, but the classic form of survey is the quantitative questionnaire sent (or handed) to an individual, with clear instructions as to how to complete and return it to the researcher. This will form the basis of this chapter.

Surveys can be carried out at one point in time, and these are termed *cross-sectional*, in that the survey is given out across an entire sample at roughly the same time, if not exactly on the same day. Cross-sectional surveys are typically *descriptive*, in that they literally describe the phenomenon of choice (for example the incidence of falls in the elderly or the incidence of side-effects caused by a drug). In addition to these target data, surveys usually contain demographic data which describe the population, for example age, gender, rank or pay band. This information can be very useful, as it allows the researcher to explore the characteristics of the different groups within the sample, which can add depth and meaning to the analysis (this will be discussed in Chapter 7). Surveys can also be *retrospective*, looking back on activities perhaps by reviewing a selection of patients' notes in a doctor's surgery.

Survey work can be extended over a period of time, the questionnaire being given out at different time intervals; this then becomes a *longitudinal survey*, which follows the progress of a population. An example could be a questionnaire exploring morale within an organisation, which is given out every year so that changes in staff attitudes can be identified over a period of time. This may also be termed an *analytic survey*, in that it analyses the changes that take place and will involve statistical analyses to identify how the population has changed and whether this is statistically significant.

What can be surveyed?

The short answer is: almost anything. Surveys are extremely flexible. If a questionnaire item can be framed that goes some way to answering the research question, then a survey can be conducted. With more items within the questionnaire, a fuller picture of the population response can be developed. As questions accumulate, the survey questionnaire begins to take shape. An important issue to consider is the provenance of these items within the questionnaire. For a questionnaire to be valid, the source of the items should be clear. They may be generated from qualitative research (such as focus groups or interviews), from background reading or from other sources. This seems obvious, but a questionnaire that can prove its provenance is likely to be robust and produce valid findings, rather than one in which the questions are thought up by the researcher in isolation.

By illustration, a small abstract painting on canvas may be attractive and fetch £50 or even £100, but if it is anonymous it is unlikely to be very valuable. With seven letters in the lower right-hand corner, it may be worth millions, particularly if they spell 'Picasso'. In addition, Fink (1995) suggests that an expert should be used to review items and Gillham (2000a) identifies that piloting is an important step to support this process.

Non-healthcare surveys can be used for political and consumer choices. Researchers can use surveys to explore feelings, motivations, plans, beliefs and perusal background (Bowling, 2009). Translated to healthcare, issues can include satisfaction with services, how services can be improved, wellbeing and health status, lifestyles and exposure to disease risk factors. With a survey, the questionnaire is the central component. It may be necessary to invest time and energy in making it easy to read, easy to use and likely to produce valid results, but once this has been done it is essentially as easy to give to 10, 100 or even 1,000 respondents. This is a very attractive proposition for researchers and goes some way to explaining the popularity of surveys.

Who can be surveyed?

In the previous chapter, it was identified that experiments largely required probability sampling to make them robust. Probability sampling is also suitable for surveys, and is generally recommend, in line with 'scientific' processes. However, surveys do not rely on their sampling in the same way, as they do not claim to identify cause and effect because association is less stringent than cause and effect (i.e. it makes fewer claims). Other strategies are available and justifiable: these may be classified as non-probability sampling and have been discussed in the previous chapter.

Cohort studies

One of the most robust forms of survey research is the cohort study. As the name suggests, in a cohort study a group of people (the cohort) are followed over a period of time. In a retrospective design, the cohort is identified and then records are searched to gather data about the topic of interest. In a prospective design, the cohort is identified and data are collected over a specified period of time, which may span days, months or years. These are non-experimental designs because there is no introduction of an intervention; however, the study may be controlled by comparison with a parallel group.

Although strictly speaking, cohort studies can only show association, in practice a well-designed prospective study can be seen as providing robust evidence that effectively shows causality. For example, in a world-famous study of the effects of tobacco smoking (known widely as 'The Doctors' Study'), Doll *et al.* (2004) completed a study that had been running for 50 years in the UK. The cohort was a group of male doctors born between 1900 and 1930, who were surveyed in 1957, 1966, 1971, 1978, 1991 and finally in 2001. Every male doctor on the UK medical practitioner register was invited to take part, yielding an initial sample of 34,439 doctors. Although the study evolved over time, the basics were clear: this was a prospective cohort controlled study – the control consisted of the doctors who did not smoke. Throughout the study, a consistent picture appeared: namely that smokers had a greater risk of both myocardial infarction and lung cancer. Although there was variation depending on the amount smoked and the period it was smoked over, the study found that smoking decreases lifespan by 10 years, and that 50% of all smokers die of a disease known to be related to smoking. This has shaped attitudes towards smoking over the last 50 years, showing the impact of this research.

Response rates

Surveys are not like experiments. There is limited control of the variables, even in a longitudinal survey. One issue that exemplifies this lack of control is response rate. A survey can be drafted, piloted and administered. Part of the ethical considerations involved in healthcare research is the issue of consent. A common way of addressing this is to assume that completion and return of the questionnaire is evidence of consent to take part. This means that it is unethical to force or pressurise participants to complete it. Commonly this means that response rates are low or at best variable, and this can introduce bias.

All surveyors would hope for a high response rate: for example, greater than 90% would be excellent. This is seldom achieved though. A response rate greater than 70% is often considered adequate. Experience has shown that amongst nurses, midwives and other healthcare professionals 50% is an achievable target, and amongst students it may be somewhat lower (for an example, see Norrie and Dalby (2007)). Exactly why this should be the case is not always clear. Within a health setting, the workers are commonly very busy and may be pressurised to complete their work on time, so filling in yet another questionnaire may reasonably be a very low priority. Similarly, paperwork in healthcare settings may itself be a burden for workers. There may be an issue of 'questionnaire fatigue.' Finally staff may be suspicious of the questionnaire, and see it possibly as a management tool. What results therefore is a bias in the return sample, which may be severe.

This does not mean that a survey should be abandoned because, for example, it only achieved a return rate of 35%; it does, however, mean that the low return rate should be acknowledged and discussed. If it is wished to utilise such a survey's findings in practice it would be wise to seek support from other research literature. Emotive topics such as domestic violence and sexual content may generate lower returns, and an unsolicited survey, where there is no prior contact with the subjects, may have a response rate of less than 20%.

To overcome this tendency for a low response rate, researchers have a number of tactics. One is to offer inducements to respond. This could include entering names into a lottery draw of some sort, but this may compromise anonymity. Another is to offer a small token of thanks, and for those working with nurses it may come as no surprise that these tokens are often in the form of chocolate!

One more formal tactic which should always be used is a clear explanation of the aims of the research, including an outline of what the practitioners or clients or service might gain from the work. This should be part of a Participant Information Sheet that accompanies the questionnaire. This should be couched in broad terms; otherwise it may influence the ways in which the questionnaires are completed.

Bearing this in mind, it is still important to have an approximate guide to the size of sample to be aimed for. Teddlie and Tashakkori (2009) use Table 6.1 to show the relationship between sample and population sizes.

Clearly the larger the sample size, the more confident we can be that the sample represents the population. Indeed, this table illustrates that with small populations it is necessary to sample the majority of the population, to be confident that the data are representative. However, as the population increases, if we use the plus or minus 5% category, which is a level of confidence that most

Table 6.1 Sample size and confidence.

Population size	Confident that the sample estimates population within plus or minus 1%	Confident that the sample estimates population within plus or minus 5%
100	99	80
500	476	218
1,000	906	278
2,000	1,656	323
3,000	2,286	341
Infinity	9,604	384

survey researchers would think advisable, there is a plateau effect: samples in the range of 300–400 appear to be broadly representative of their populations. If the sample size increases above these values, then the researchers reduce the amount of variance from the true population, but the extent to which this is achieved then becomes a matter of resources.

Two caveats are necessary. Firstly, this table is predicated upon using a probability sampling technique. Therefore it holds with inclusive sampling, but if non-probability samplings such as purposive strategies are used the statistics should be approached with caution. Secondly, it does not address response rates. If a target of 350 responses is the goal, then a generous margin should be incorporated to optimise the chances of getting this total, for example by distributing at least 700 questionnaires, assuming a 50% return rate. Furthermore, in data analysis of surveys it is often desirable to explore differences between groups using inferential statistics, so there may be a need for power analysis, as discussed in Chapter 5.

How to construct and code a quantitative survey

Surveys commonly start or finish with a section of demographic data. This section gives information about who is completing the survey. Demographic items can include age, gender, ethnicity, clinical band, qualifications and how long respondents have been in post or within the speciality. These serve to summarise the population, but they also are useful in the application of inferential statistics, where one group is compared with another to see if there is a real difference in experience. For example, if you are exploring violence and aggression in a clinical area, it seems likely that women and men will have different experiences, or that exposure to these may be influenced by ethnicity.

There are a number of choices available of items within the survey proper. As this is a discussion of quantitative research methods, qualitative items will not be explored, although there is a role for these too (see later).

In quantitative surveys, the data produced will at some point be coded and entered into a database. This may be a familiar program such as Microsoft Excel, or a dedicated statistical package such as SPSS. SPSS is probably, on a worldwide basis, the most commonly used package in universities. One strategy is to enter data directly into Excel, which is widely available as part of Microsoft Office, and when all the data are prepared they are cut and pasted, or directly imported, into SPSS. In a quantitative survey most items are closed questions or statements. This means that there are a limited number of responses. These responses are allocated a number during coding and the numbers entered into the database. Here is an example from a piece of research looking at exposure to violence and aggression:

How often have you felt uncomfortable/threatened/unsafe due to aggression in your workplace?

- ❏ Never
- ❏ Seldom
- ❏ Occasionally
- ❏ Regularly
- ❏ Most days

The responses are coded from 1 to 5, so if the box 'Occasionally' has been ticked, then a '3' is recorded. If the box 'Never' has been ticked, a '1' is given. For data such as these which contain a scale, it is common to make coding intuitive: this means that as the likelihood of being threatened increases, so does the score given to it. Coding therefore funnels the information so that a questionnaire is summarised by a string of numbers, which can then be statistically analysed.

There a number of different levels of data that can be included in a questionnaire. In general, the higher the level of data that can be used, the better, as it provides more information and can allow more detailed analyses to be carried out (Anthony, 1999). One final note: 'data' is a plural; the singular is 'datum'.

Nominal or categorical data

These are the lowest forms of data. With nominal data there is no ordering to the information. They typically provide yes or no responses. Examples include:

- Are you pregnant?
- Do you have a previous history of hypertension?
- Were you provided with medications on discharge?

Here is another example:

Is your pain:

- ❏ Flickering
- ❏ Throbbing
- ❏ Tingling
- ❏ Crushing

There are choices here, but there is no order to the information. My pain may be tingling, but that does not mean it is more or less uncomfortable than a crushing or flickering pain. Another obvious example is gender; people on the whole are male or female. However, even here there may be some contention. If the study were to be set in a gender reassignment clinic this might need some re-working as a questionnaire item. In this circumstance it may be better to use a more flexible way of measuring to what extent a client feels male or female, perhaps on a scale from 0–10. This then produces data with an order to them, termed ordinal data.

Ordinal data

With ordinal data, there is an order but not a fixed relationship between points. A good example of ordinal data is the numbering of motorway junctions. Between London and Leicester there are 21 junctions on the M1 (we ignore later additions, such as junction 15A, for simplicity). When map reading, these can be ticked off and it is straightforward to identify that there are 3, 6 or 10 junctions to go, which is very useful for navigation. However, the distance between motorway junctions can vary widely, from one to two miles (junctions 2–3) to more than 10 miles (junctions 20–21). The order is fixed, but the distance between points varies. Another example is swimmers finishing in a race. Giving the order (first, second, third) gives important information, but does not indicate by how much the race was won. Ordinal data are very widespread in healthcare research, particularly in quantitative surveys. Two common types are discussed below.

Likert scales

These were first developed by a North American social researcher, Rensis Likert (pronounced Lick-urt) in the 1930s. Most people will be familiar with a Likert scale questionnaire, as they are widely used in marketing and research, and have been for the last 80 years.

A statement is made, and the respondent is invited to tick one pre-formatted series of boxes which corresponds with their level of agreement. One issue of note here is that although included within a questionnaire, Likert items are not actually questions! A range of options are possible; perhaps the most common is the five-interval scale:

(1) Strongly disagree (2) Disagree (3) Neutral (4) Agree (5) Strongly agree

Rensis Likert 1903–1981 (By kind permission of Institute for Social Research of the University of Michigan)

There are variants of this, a common one being a four-item scale where the neutral category is omitted, forcing respondents to choose between being positive or negative in response. Oppenheim (1992) gives a very detailed discussion of the options available in the design and usage of Likert scales.

Visual analogue scales (VAS)

These are probably familiar to most health workers who assess client reactions. Respondents are asked to describe their pain using a visual scale to represent experiences such as pain or wellbeing.

Example: On a scale from 0–10 I would describe my pain as:

0	5	10
Nil		Severe

Strictly the client would indicate the level of their pain on the scale, and this would then be measured as the distance from the zero (this is the analogy), but in practice commonly a verbal score is given. Either way produces good-quality ordinal data which can be analysed in exactly the same way as Likert scales.

Being creative with ordinal scales

One very useful aspect of using scales is that they may not require words at all. Figure 6.1 is an example used by David Dalby of De Montfort University, exploring the satisfaction of clients with a Learning Disability with their service. It has some of the characteristics of a Likert item and some of a VAS.

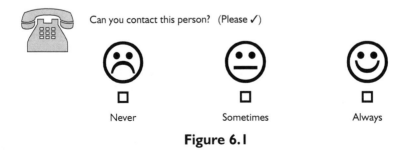

Figure 6.1

How clients use it will vary, as does the extent of disability, but one way would be to read the question out to the client, and ask them to identify which of the 'faces' they would identify with. This ability to be creative is very attractive and can lead to new and exciting methods (Grbich, 2004).

The Oucher scale

Similarly, the Oucher scale was produced to measure pain in small children who could not effectively vocalise how they felt. It consists of a scale with six pictures of small children, progressing from an apparently pain-free unconcerned child, through to a clearly distressed and very unhappy one; these are real pictures taken from clinical practice. This is immediately adjacent to a percentage scale, with the former rated at 0%, through to the latter rated at 100%. The first picture is scored by giving it a value of 0, the second of 1 and so on to a maximum of 5. Alternatively, if the child is capable, a percentage score can be used. Versions of the scale are available for different ethnicities, including white, African-American and Hispanic (Peden and Saddington, 2001). An example of how to score and analyse interval level data is given in Chapter 7.

Interval level data

With interval level data, the distance between items on the scale is constant. A car travelling at 30 mph is definitely travelling at half the speed of a car at 60 mph. Interval level data are used less frequently in research that explores beliefs and subjective responses. Thus if a questionnaire is being constructed to explore patient satisfaction, it may be that only some minor items such as demographic data, particularly age or length of service, may be interval data. However, there are important uses for interval level data, especially (but not only) in medical research:

- Length of time of survival following myocardial infarction
- Number of weeks gestation
- Optimal dosages of drug for medical conditions
- Age at first pregnancy
- Patient's oral temperature following administration of paracetamol

The attraction of interval data is that they are cited as being a prerequisite for a number of important statistical techniques (which include the tests that classically analyse the outcomes of experiments) and many other techniques that are used in statistical modelling. These techniques are robust, and there are a number of researchers who successfully apply these statistical analyses to larger sets of ordinal data as long as they meet certain criteria, which will be discussed in the next chapter.

Developing a questionnaire using ordinal data

Here is an example of a Likert scale item, which the reader has already met:

	Strongly disagree	Disagree	Neutral	Agree	Strongly agree
I understand a lot about quantitative research					

Which box would you now tick? Hopefully, some readers will have increased their scores since the start of these chapters (perhaps not).

Trying to sum up a response to quite a complex topic such as the world of quantitative research with a one-item questionnaire would be unwise. As you may have discovered, there are lots of different topics within quantitative research methods. Some are actually quite straightforward, others definitely not so. How could one question encompass the lot?

Here is another example. If I were to invite a number of friends to my house for their evening meal, as a quantitative researcher (there is after all no such thing as a free lunch), I might produce a questionnaire to see how much they enjoyed it. I have a number of options:

- *Using nominal data* I am quite limited: did you enjoy the meal? The responses could be only yes or no, which provides me with limited information.
- *Using ordinal data* is better: I could make a statement 'The meal was excellent' and put it in a Likert scale format (Strongly disagree → Strongly agree). This would be better, but it ignores the fact that a good meal is made up of a number of items, some of which may have been good, others awful.

- *Use of a single score* is too crude: it cannot tell if there are different factors to be explored. In addition, one poorly constructed question may ruin the survey entirely.

It would be more sensitive to identify a number of items that might describe the experience of the meal: for example, the size of the portions, the quality of the wines which accompanied it, how well seasoned it was etc. This results in a bank of Likert items, all of which relate to the meal. Taken overall each item contributes to the overall assessment of the quality of the meal, and each contributes its own unique quality.

On p. 109 is an example of part of a questionnaire (there were originally 12 items, which have been edited down) used in a research project to explore the ways in which student nurses identify their learning styles (adapted from Norrie and Dalby 2007).

Discussion: The first item is a set of demographic questions, identifying the year of studies, nursing branch and programme. This allows us to summarise who the respondents are, and specifically who has completed the questionnaire. These data can also be used to see if there are differences in response according to any of these criteria, so as to compare groups. Techniques for doing this will be discussed in the next chapter. The second item is a bank of Likert scale items, which all explore different aspects of ways in which the student nurses learn, based upon focus group work. If all the items score consistently high, or low, then the questionnaire is said to be internally reliable, which is a hallmark of good quality.

Including qualitative elements in a survey

Finally, although this chapter has discussed quantitative questionnaires, there is still a place for some qualitative work. Coming from a deductive methodology produces a possible weakness. The questionnaire was produced, following focus groups with nurse lecturers, to identify the issues which they felt were important. However, this is not to say that *all* the important issues were included. Therefore it is a common strategy of quantitative researchers to include a small number of open-ended questions to identify inductively any items that may have been missed from the questionnaire which are of importance to the respondents.

Part A: Identify and categorise the different components used.
Which year of your studies are you in:

Year 1 ❑
Year 2 ❑
Year 3 ❑

1. Which branch are you in?
Mental Health ❑
Learning Disability ❑
Child ❑
Adult ❑

2. Are you undertaking a:
Degree ❑
Diploma ❑

Part B: For each item, please tick one box only which best describes your opinion

	Strongly agree	Agree	Disagree	Strongly disagree
It is important to me to know which subjects I need to learn				
I prefer to manage my own learning				
I seldom add to my learning with independent study				
I like to be thoroughly prepared before starting a module				
I like to be taught rather than finding out on my own				
I do not find exploring the experiences of others is a good way of learning				
I like to know why it is important to learn a topic				

Part C: In your own words, can you briefly identify the best methods which help you learn?

Alpha analysis

This is assessed by using a statistical test called an alpha analysis (Field, 2009). The highest possible alpha score is 1.0. This would mean that each item gave essentially identical responses, meaning that the questionnaire was asking the same question (in this case) seven times. If the alpha value is low (for example 0.2), then the questions are identifying a number of different issues within the responses. In this case, individual items would be investigated and reported.

With a moderately high alpha (greater than 0.7–0.8) it is usually safe to summate the scale. This means that the responses for each item can be added up and an overall average score take. This then represents the body of the questionnaire, and is much more dependable than asking one question.

Commercial and pre-validated questionnaires

A wide range of questionnaires have been developed to explore aspects of psychology and wellbeing. The benefit of these is that they have been used over years and often decades. Previous workers have found them to be reliable and valid, and a substantial literature has grown up around them, so that they are widely accepted as being robust. Four examples will be introduced here: SF-36 (Short Form 36), EQ-5D (EuroQol 5 Dimensions), HADS (Hospital Anxiety and Depression Score) and EPDS. All the questionnaires consist of a range of ordinal items.

SF-36

As the name suggests, there are 36 questions in the SF-36 questionnaire. It is administered by a private company, Quality Metric (2013). The questions cover eight dimensions: physical functioning, role – physical, bodily pain, general health, vitality, social functioning, role – emotional and mental health. Each of these subscales can be reported independently, or as two scores, one for physical and one for mental health, or as an overall score. It can be administered electronically, in an interview situation or as a paper questionnaire. It is available in most languages. Here is an example of items which explore how health issues may impact on the participants' activities:

During the past 4 weeks, how much of the time have you had any of the following problems with your work or other regular daily activities as a result of your physical health?

	All of the time	Most of the time	Some of the time	A little of the time	None of the time
Cut down on the amount of time you spent on work or other activities	❑	❑	❑	❑	❑
Accomplished less than you would like	❑	❑	❑	❑	❑
Were limited in the kind of work or other activities	❑	❑	❑	❑	❑

The responses from the questionnaire are summed and transformed to give a score between 0 and 100. As can be seen from the subscales, it is generic in that it is not aimed at any particular age group or health condition. It has been used in over 4,000 publications. Shorter versions of it are available; SF-12 (i.e. 12 questions) is now available as an application for smartphones. The questionnaires can only be used under license, and the licenses have to be paid for.

EQ-5D

The EuroQol group is a commercial body which developed this questionnaire. As with SF-36, it is a generic measure of wellbeing and again payment is required before use. The current version is the EQ-5D-5L, which uses a five-point ordinal scale to cover five dimensions of health: mobility, self-care, usual activities, pain/discomfort and anxiety/depression. Here is an example of one dimension, 'mobility', with its associated tick boxes:

I have no problems in walking about ❑
I have slight problems in walking about ❑
I have moderate problems in walking about ❑
I have severe problems in walking about ❑
I am unable to walk about ❑

In addition, the questionnaire uses a 0–100 visual analogue scale to give an overall score of health. In the UK the score is the preferred measure of generic health used by the National Institute for Health and Clinical Excellence (NICE) (2008), although Bowling (2009, p. 116) identifies a number of weaknesses, describing it as lacking response to some conditions (e.g. visual problems) and of being 'relatively crude'. In general EQ-5D is used mainly in Europe.

HADS

The Hospital Anxiety and Depression Score was produced in 1983 by Zigmond and Snaith, who undertook research in a general medical setting. As the name suggests, it measures two dimensions: anxiety and depression. Each is represented by seven questions, which means that the HADS can easily be presented as a single sheet of A4 paper; it thus has the value of brevity. Two items are shown below, with their scoring:

A	I feel tense or 'wound up':	
	Most of the time	3
	A lot of the time	2
	From time to time	I
	Not at all	0
D	I still enjoy the things I used to enjoy:	
	Definitely as much	3
	Not quite as much	2
	Only a little	I
	Hardly at all	0

Bjelland *et al.* (2002) reviewed 747 publications which had used HADS and concluded that it performed well in assessing both anxiety and depression. It was found that a score of eight or more for either subscale was a suitable cut-off to identify anxiety and or depression. HADS has been used widely in medicine and surgery, including end-stage renal failure, brain injury, cancer and palliative care. It is thus very widely accepted. It is available commercially from GL Assessment via their website; payment would be necessary for a research project to use HADS.

EPDS

The Edinburgh Postnatal Depression Score was produced by Cox *et al.* in 1987 and is used widely in the USA and UK. It is designed to be used by women within the eight weeks following birth, or as a pre-natal assessment. It consists of 10 ordinal scale statements (Andrews-Fike, 1999). Here are two examples:

I have been able to laugh and see the funny side of things
- ❏ As much as I always could
- ❏ Not quite so much now
- ❏ Definitely not as much now
- ❏ Not at all

I have looked forward with enjoyment to things
- ❏ As much as I ever did
- ❏ Rather less than I used to
- ❏ Definitely less than I used to
- ❏ Hardly at all

As with the HADS, this scale has the great advantage of being presented on a single sheet of A4, and is very quick to complete, analyse and interpret. EPDS scores are simply added up. A score above a threshold of 12–13 is seen as indicating potential depressive symptoms which might be suggestive of post-partum depression. In the UK, it has been recommended by NICE in their Clinical Guideline 45 for use with women, following birth, who are considered to be at risk of post-partum depression, following an initial assessment (as indeed is the HADS) (NICE, 2007).

These are four examples of pre-validated scales. The first two (SF-36, EQ-5D), are generic, giving an overview of general health. The latter two are specific, measuring two aspects of mental health, namely depression (HADS and EDPS) and anxiety (HADS). There are many other scales available. An informal Internet search (early 2013) reveals scales to measure depression, hopelessness, anxiety, phobias, binge eating, aggression and many, many more aspects of health and personality. The significance of using scales such as these is that they are often used to measure health states in a research context. For example, the use of kyphoplasty to treat vertebral compression aims to improve overall quality of mobility and other aspects of life, including reduction in pain and improvement of breathing. It involves injection of cement into collapsed vertebrae. A randomised controlled trial by Buchbinder *et al.* (2010) used EQ-5D to compare the intervention group (injection of cement) against the control of best conventional therapy, whilst another study (Kallmes *et al.*, 2009) used SF-36. Because repeated use and academic study have confirmed that these have both validity and reliability, they can be used with confidence in high-quality studies. Interestingly, neither study found significant differences with regard to placebo.

Ways to improve a survey

The survey should always be piloted before use. Drawing up a questionnaire is fairly easy. However, the researcher may be oblivious to a number of faults within it, even though to him or her it may seem clear and unambiguous. The problem is that the author is always biased, having created it, and may have lost objective perspective. This may threaten its validity. Common issues which are found include:

- Are the questions unambiguous?
- Can respondents understand the language and terminology?

To address these issues, it is usual to pilot the questionnaire with a group of respondents similar to the intended one in the final survey, but who are not *actually* in it. If carrying out a survey of community midwives, then it might be reasonable to pilot the questionnaire with a group of community midwives in a different Trust, or a similar group in another geographical area. The idea here is to avoid introducing bias into the sample group by pre-exposure to the questionnaire, or in layman's terms 'muddying the water'. This process is always extremely valuable, and it is common to find that even (in the researcher's mind) the most straightforward questions can be open to a number of interpretations, which will threaten the validity of the research. The pilot group does not have to be a large one, and as few as 10–12 individuals will do, as long as their comments and suggestions are heeded and included in the final questionnaire. By this process it is common for the questionnaire to go through a number of developmental stages before finalisation, but this step is always necessary and essential.

CHAPTER 7

Quantitative research: data analysis

Statistics is the branch of mathematics that deals with collecting, organizing and interpreting data using systematic procedures. Surprisingly, it aims to simplify the data, not complicate them. Experience has shown that nurses and midwives, on the whole, are reluctant statisticians; however, it is equally likely that statisticians would probably make terrible carers. It is also true that statistics can be very, very complicated. Fortunately the use of computers and statistical software packages has taken a lot of the hard work out of quantitative data analysis. Most people who have a computer run Microsoft Windows software. If you also have Microsoft Office, then you will have a copy of Microsoft Excel. This can be used to explore data, and although Excel is widely used for fairly simple tasks, such as keeping household budgets, it can be used in much more exciting ways. In this chapter it will be used to explore some examples of both descriptive and inferential statistics, to get the reader to interact with some data.

Most students who get involved with statistics in some way will want a more specialised tool and there are a number available. SPSS is one of these, and is widely used in the UK and USA. There are a number of guides for using it, and the best of these include data sets on CD or available online, so that students can not only read about what to do, but actually do it in real time. Two good examples are written by Argyrous (2005) and Field (2009). The former is an excellent starting point and would be likely to be adequate for degree and masters level work. Once you have been bitten by the bug and cannot stop, then Field's book will give you all the detail that you will ever need, and is the only book on statistical data analysis (so far) which is likely to make the reader laugh out loud.

Entering data in Excel

The examples here use the 2007 version of Excel. Earlier ones are very similar, but may take a little flexibility on behalf of the user.

When Excel is opened up, the main page is presented as a set of cells. Entering data is fairly straightforward; clicking on a cell allows the entry of data in either the cell itself, or in the function dialogue box:

Here are two sets of data, developed from an exercise I have used with Learning Beyond Registration healthcare degree students.

Data set A is the heart rate of the students before a coffee break, when both their spirits and their physiology have been depressed listening to an interminable lecture on survey research. Set B is the same set of students immediately after a coffee break, when suitably loaded up with caffeine and/or nicotine they have returned to the lecture.

Now do Excel exercise 1.

This chapter will introduce two main types of statistics: descriptive and inferential. It is always best to do the descriptive work first, followed by the inferential.

Descriptive statistics

These literally describe the population, so that a set of numbers can be described and summarised. Descriptive statistics are the essential first step in data analysis and although relatively straightforward are very valuable. Examples include:

- Frequencies, percentages, measures of central tendency; these are all numerical ways to present data.
- Tables, charts; these are graphical ways to present data.

For a survey they may be the only statistics required. Commonly, however, it is desirable or necessary to go further, for example to compare one population with another; the classic example would be for an experiment in which it is necessary to compare values for two sets of dependent variables. Techniques such as these are termed inferential statistics.

Excel exercise I

Enter the following data into Excel, plus the titles at the foot of the columns. The data should then look like this:

	Group A	Group B
	80	77
	89	86
	78	76
	76	99
	68	74
	92	67
	87	83
	93	87
	83	85
	84	87
	82	81
	84	89
	78	71
	86	95
	74	90
	77	96
	73	86
	96	92
	71	81
	64	79
Max		
Min		
Average		
Median		
Mode		
Sdev		
t test		

Inferential statistics

These provide predictions about populations. They do more than describe data; they can predict behaviour between variables. Examples, which will be discussed later, include *t*-tests, **Analysis of Variance**, **Mann–Whitney** and **Kruskal–Wallis** tests.

Descriptive statistics: what do the data look like?

Do not underestimate the power of descriptive statistics. They are a necessary first step and allow you to engage meaningfully with the data.

Tables

Tables are commonly used to summarise frequencies, i.e. to count the number of cases in which a variable occurs. Table 7.1 is an example of a table from SPSS.

The variable is the marks for a research module. The frequency is the number of students who scored that particular mark. The other headings are of less interest: the differences between Percent and Valid percent are caused by missing data, and the cumulative total always adds up to 100% of the cases. This is a good example of SPSS output, in that not only does it give you the data you need, it also gives you quite a lot of content you do not.

Just doing this has helped display the data so that we can see the lowest, or minimum score (35%) and the highest or maximum (80%). In addition, we can see that there are higher frequencies between 52–60%, so we might expect the average score to be in this range:

Now do Excel exercise 2.

Table 7.1 Example of SPSS table output.

Marks as %

		Frequency	Percent	Valid Percent	Cumulative Percent
Valid	35	1	1.0	1.2	1.2
	40	5	5.2	5.9	7.1
	42	2	2.1	2.4	9.4
	43	4	4.2	4.7	14.1
	45	5	5.2	5.9	20.0
	46	1	1.0	1.2	21.2
	48	2	2.1	2.4	23.5
	49	1	1.0	1.2	24.7
	50	3	3.1	3.5	28.2
	51	1	1.0	1.2	29.4
	52	7	7.3	8.2	37.6
	55	6	6.2	7.1	44.7
	56	3	3.1	3.5	48.2
	58	11	11.5	12.9	61.2
	60	3	3.1	3.5	64.7
	61	1	1.0	1.2	65.9
	62	7	7.3	8.2	74.1
	63	1	1.0	1.2	75.3
	64	1	1.0	1.2	76.5
	65	4	4.2	4.7	81.2
	66	1	1.0	1.2	82.4
	68	6	6.2	7.1	89.4
	71	1	1.0	1.2	90.6
	72	6	6.2	7.1	97.6
	75	1	1.0	1.2	98.8
	80	1	1.0	1.2	100.0
	Total	85	88.5	100.0	
Missing	System	11	11.5		
Total		96	100.0		

Excel exercise 2

As we have seen, a first step in exploring the Excel data is to put them in order. To do this, click and drag over the numbers in data set A; if you are unsure how to do this, ask any teenager! The spreadsheet will look like this:

Group A	Group B
80	77
89	86
78	76
76	99
68	74
92	67
87	83
93	87
83	85
84	87
82	81
84	89
78	71
86	95
74	90
77	96
73	86
96	92
71	81
64	79

Now go to the 'sort and filter' command on the taskbar at the top of the page. Click on the little arrow on the bottom right and you will be presented with a number of options. Click on the first 'Sort Smallest to Largest'; this will sort the table for you, so you can inspect the data, as we did for the marks table. Ignore invitations to 'expand the data', and opt to continue with the current selection.

The table should now look like this:

Group A	Group B
64	77
68	80
71	76
73	99
74	74
76	67
77	83
78	87
78	85
80	87
82	81
83	89
84	71
84	95
86	90
87	96
89	86
92	92
93	81
96	79

Repeat the process for group B. Start to get a feel for the data. Are the maximums and minimums similar or different? Input the values for maximum and minimum on the Excel spreadsheet.

Max	96	99
Min	64	67
Average		
Median		
Mode		
Sdeviation		
t test		

Where is the middle of the range? Having inspected the data, you may come to some conclusions as to where this lies, but it should already be obvious that more detail is necessary to explore even these small sets of data.

This exercise has shown that tables can be useful to summarise a set of data. It is unusual to display tables of a data set in a publication, as they are quite cumbersome; instead, charts may provide a more visual and readily accessible summary.

Charts

There are many different types of chart. Three commonly used are:

- Bar charts
- Histograms
- Pie charts

Bar chart

Having spent some time extolling the virtues of Excel, we will take one step back – Excel is good, but the graphics package which comes with it is not very flexible. Instead, for this section SPSS will be used to display examples of data.

Bar charts are one of the simplest charts. They are used to display nominal and ordinal data. Typically, the nominal variable is entered on the horizontal (or x) axis, to represent the grouping of the data, and the frequency of cases (if categorical) or mean values (if ordinal or interval) are represented by the vertical (or y) axis.

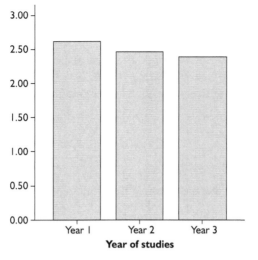

Figure 7.1 Example of a bar chart.

This is taken from Norrie and Dalby (2007). In this study 318 pre-registration nursing students completed a survey, using a set of Likert scale statements, to explore their preferred ways of learning. The *y*-axis represents their willingness to manage their own learning and uses the average value (or mean, to be mathematically more accurate). The *x*-axis is grouped in three increments to show their year of study. This bar chart seems to show that as the students progressed through their studies, their scores decreased; this shows that they become more reluctant to manage their own learning, and hence behaved less like adult learners; a trait which was picked up by other statements in the questionnaire. A lot of data have therefore been usefully summarised here, so that a clear message has been produced. This does, however, need to be explored further, using both descriptive and inferential statistics.

Histograms

Histograms are similar, but they are used where the data on the *x*-axis are continuous, so they should be interval. With a histogram, the data are grouped into blocks, so that each bar represents a range of data; in this example, each block represents a value of two marks.

Figure 7.2 is another set of marks, from yet another research module. This is clearly a superior way of looking at the data, compared to a table. Here it can be seen that the main grouping lies between 58% and 66%, but that there is another grouping between 44% and 50%. This is, however, open to interpretation (is there also a high scoring group?) and illustrates again that showing the data in a chart, although very useful, has its limitations.

Pie chart

A pie chart is a circle that has been partitioned into percentage groups of nominal or ordinal variables. It is a very clear way of providing an overview of the population. If there are more than six variables it may become too cluttered (Munro, 2005).

Here is an example taken from a Masters Degree project, which was subsequently published (Norrie, 1997). In this research, nurses working in an Intensive Cardiothoracic Unit were asked to log how they spent their time, at the end of each hour, using five activity descriptors. Figure 7.3 shows these data as a pie chart.

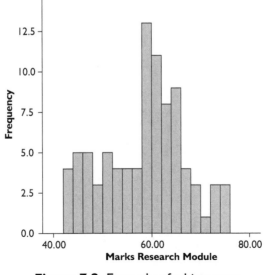

Figure 7.2 Example of a histogram.

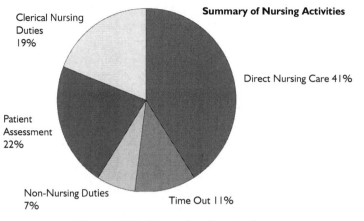

Figure 7.3 Example of a pie chart.

The pie chart shows clearly that the majority of their time was spent working in appropriate activities; three slices of the pie, Direct Nursing Care, Patient Assessment and Clerical Nursing Duties together add up to 82% of the nurses' time, and these figures were used to support the nursing management structures used at that time.

Box plots

The final chart to be explored is the box plot. These are useful because they clearly show differences between populations. They are based upon the use of percentiles.

The box plot in Figure 7.4 (overleaf) is part of the results from a research project exploring the achievement of students in an English university during their nursing diplomas and degrees (Dyson *et al.*, 2008).

There are two groups shown for comparison. One is 'Other', representing non-Asian students (a mix of predominantly white and smaller numbers of black students), and the other group contains students who described themselves as 'Asian' (primarily second generation students from the Indian sub-continent). The average marks for their studies over a period of three years are shown on the left side. The chart shows:

- **The median**: this is the bar in the middle of the boxes. It is a measurement of central tendency, and is one way to summarise what the main characteristic of the population is. In everyday terms we might describe this as an 'average' (although, as will be shown, this is not strictly correct). If you look closely at the median values, it can be seen that the 'Other' group has a slightly higher value than the 'Asian' group suggesting that they get slightly better marks overall.

- **The boxes**: the shaded area above the medians shows where the first 25% of the population above the median lie, and the shaded area below shows where the first 25% of the population below the median lie. These are termed percentiles, and will be familiar to any health professional who deals with growth and development in children. Thus the first 50% of the population is summarised within the boxes.

- **The tails**: populations spread out from the central values, and the tails pick up the remaining 25% above and 25% below the 50% grouping. There are a number of outliers (which have data set numbers attached to them, so that we can check they have been entered correctly); these are values which SPSS has identified as falling outside of the main population and as being 'odd'.

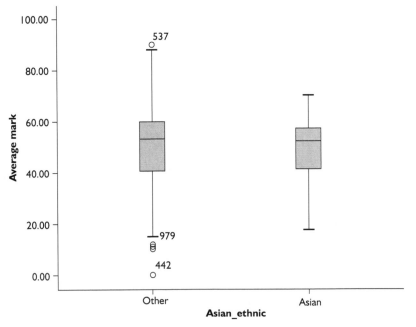

Figure 7.4 Example of a box plot.

The box plot allows us to compare the two groups. Basically they look quite similar, but both the median and first 25% above the median of the 'Other' grouping are slightly higher, so as a first step in analysis it may be thought that the 'Other' students do slightly better than the 'Asian' ones. What this does not show is whether this is a real difference which can be used with confidence to predict future outcomes. To do this it is necessary to use statistics to explore the group. Now do Excel exercise 3.

Excel exercise 3

Figure 7.5 shows the box plots for the Excel heart rate data: what can you tell from them? Does it make a case for a difference between populations, and if so, which group has the higher values?

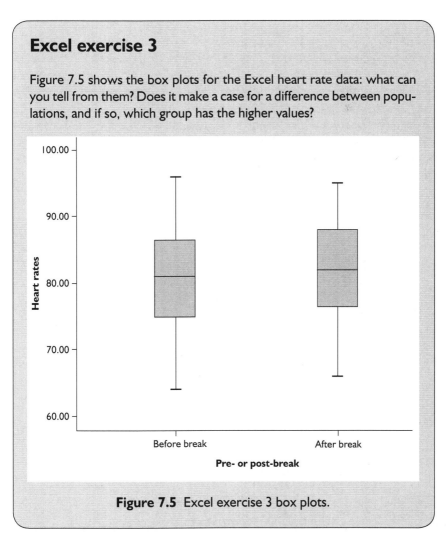

Figure 7.5 Excel exercise 3 box plots.

In summary, although tables can be a useful preliminary to sorting and inspecting data sets, the use of charts further simplifies and illustrates the process. Even so, charts have limitations and it is necessary to start to use statistical techniques to explore the information hidden in the numbers.

Looking at populations

Charts allow us to inspect the data we are interested in. Here are the histograms for the Excel data, entered into SPSS. SPSS has overlaid a very characteristic shape on the charts using a curved black line. This classic symmetrical bell-shaped curve is termed the normal (or parametric) population. Figures 7.6 and 7.7 show the histograms for populations A and B.

The characteristic shape of the normal population is important because if the data correspond to a normal population (i.e. can honestly be described as being approximately 'normal'), then a number of predictions can be made. This is important in statistical analysis.

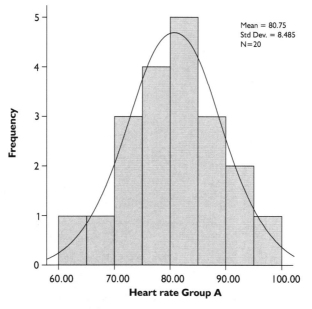

Figure 7.6 Histogram of data set A.

A normal population:

- Has a characteristic bell-shaped curve
- Is symmetrical
- Encompasses almost all the data set
  Now do Excel exercise 4 (overleaf).

Terminology

Most text books describe this characteristic bell-shaped curve as being 'normal'. If the population does not fit this shape it is commonly said to be 'not normal'. There is a problem here for researchers interested in healthcare, where we try to be inclusive. There is an inference that subjects who do not fit within the normal distribution are (by extension) 'not normal'. For example, if we are exploring intelligence, then a small number of people will always fall outside the normal distribution, but it is ugly terminology to describe them as being 'not normal'. This sort of terminology was used by the eugenic movement in the early 20th

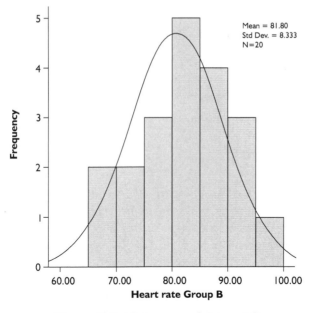

Figure 7.7 Histogram of data set B.

Excel exercise 4

Review the histograms for the two populations. Do they look normal? Justify your decision.

Analysis

Inspection of charts such as these is one way of assessing whether a population follows the normal distribution. There is a problem, however, because for statisticians it is quite desirable for their population to be normal, as this allows advanced statistical techniques to be used. This means there is a possibility of bias, and it has been shown that people who publish healthcare research tend to make this assumption, often without justification (Anthony, 1996). For the statistically minded, the Kolmogorov–Smirnov test (available in SPSS, but not Excel) can be applied to the data to give a much more robust estimate. Using it for both these sets of data, it can be confirmed that they are indeed normally distributed.

century, which had totally abhorrent views on race that are not acceptable in the 21st. There is, fortunately, an alternative. The normal population can also be said to be *parametric*, which means that it adheres to the parameters or characteristics identified above. Populations which do not conform to these parameters are said to be *non-parametric*, and these are the terms that will be used from now on.

Central tendency

So far, we have reviewed a number of ways to get a feel for data. It is now necessary to be more precise. Researchers are commonly interested in the idea of measuring the central tendency of a population. This is the number that best summarises the main body of the data. In everyday usage we might say that 'on average' I drink 20 units of alcohol per week, or smoke 20 cigarettes per day. Clearly, when exploring data sets, it is necessary to be more precise than this. There are three main ways to represent central tendency: average or mean, median and mode.

■ **Average or mean**

The mean is the true mathematical average of the population. To calculate this, all the values in a population are added together and divided by the number of cases. The mean is probably the most widely accepted and understood measure of central tendency, but it has limitations. It can be affected by a small number of extreme scores. For this reason it works well with a parametric population, but should be treated with some caution in a non-parametric one.

■ **Median**

This is the middle value of a set of ordered numbers. Imagine that we have 21 people in a room, and we arrange them in a line so that the smallest is on one end and the tallest on the other end. The person who is in the middle is the median. 10 people will be taller (50% of the population will lie above the median) and 10 will be shorter (50% of the population will lie below the median). In fact, with this small set of data, there are some inconsistencies (having chosen one person as the median, this then reduces the percentage above and below), but in practice this is not a problem, as most data sets are much larger. Similarly, if there are an even number people in the data set, the value between the two mid-points can be calculated (so it is quite common to have a median with a value plus or minus 0.5). This method is much more resistant to extreme cases than the mean and so is commonly used with non-parametric populations.

■ **Mode**

This is the simplest of all measures of central tendency. It is not calculated at all, it is spotted. It is the most frequent value or category in a data set. Some non-parametric populations, far from having an elegant bell-shaped distribution, are decidedly lumpy, and so may have a number of peaks or modes; these are described as multimodal distributions. Now do Excel exercise 5.

Excel exercise 5

Excel can be used to identify the three measures of central tendency. Click on the cell next to 'average'; this tells the computer where you want the results to be delivered.

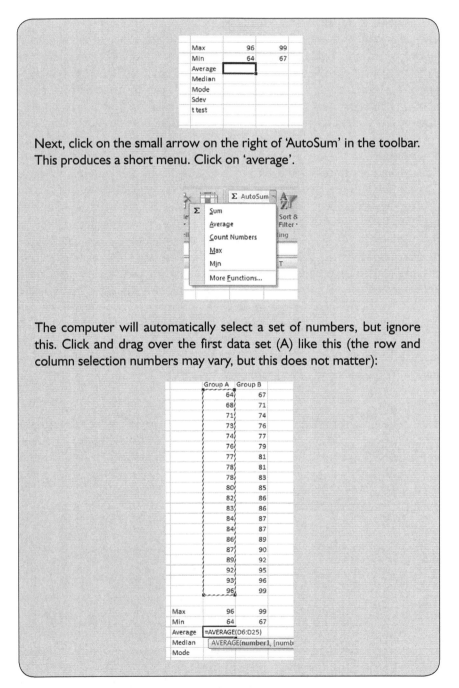

Next, click on the small arrow on the right of 'AutoSum' in the toolbar. This produces a short menu. Click on 'average'.

The computer will automatically select a set of numbers, but ignore this. Click and drag over the first data set (A) like this (the row and column selection numbers may vary, but this does not matter):

Now press 'Enter' on your keyboard, and the average will appear!

Max	96	99
Min	64	67
Average	80.75	
Median		
Mode		
Sdev		
t test		

This is the basic technique for running samples in Excel, so it is worth getting your technique perfect. Work out the average for group B.

Medians and modes are found by using the same technique; click on the space for the median for set A. It is now necessary to go into the AutoSum command, as before, and click on the 'More Functions' tab. A dialogue box appears and you can then type 'Median' in the 'Search for a Function' window.

Insert Function

Search for a function:

median — **Go**

Or select a category: Most Recently Used

Select a function:

STDEV
SUM
AVERAGE
IF
HYPERLINK
COUNT
MAX

STDEV(number1,number2,...)
Estimates standard deviation based on a sample (ignores logical values and text in the sample).

Help on this function — OK — Cancel

Click on 'Go', and repeat the process of highlighting the individual data sets. Once highlighted, click on 'OK'. The computer will automatically select the data it thinks you want to analyse, but it is always better to select your own (it does have some strange ideas at times). Repeat for set B and to find the modes for both sets. Your table should now look like this:

Max	96	99
Min	64	67
Average	80.75	84.05
Median	81	85.5
Mode	78	81
Sdev		
t test		

This a good time to compare the means, medians and modes. We already know that these populations are parametric; therefore the mean is the main indicator of central tendency that we should use. The mean in set B is higher, suggesting that the students had higher heart rates following their coffee break. This finding is supported by examination of the median and mode, which show a similar difference. One final characteristic of a parametric distribution is that the mean, median and mode are very similar, or even identical.

Standard deviation

The data so far seem to indicate that group B has a higher heart rate than group A, but before accepting this we need some more information.

Standard deviation (SD) measures the spread of a population. If we wish to compare populations, we not only need to know the measure of central tendency, but we also need to know how far the population spreads above and below the mean. This is calculated by subtracting each variable from the mean, following which the result is squared, summed and divided by the number of individuals in the population. The square root of this value is then taken. Ideally SD should only be used in populations which are parametric (but they do crop up elsewhere). Now do Excel exercise 6.

Excel exercise 6

We can calculate SD using Excel. As before, click on the cell where you wish the data to be recorded for group A's SD.

Max	96	99
Min	64	67
Average	80.75	84.05
Median	81	85.5
Mode	78	81
Sdev		
t test		

Next click on the little triangular tab at the right of the AutoSum box. It will show some options:

Click on More Functions. A dialogue box will come up. You can either look through the various menus, or simply type in STDEV (as shown below), then click Go.

The computer will actually present you with a number of slightly different ways to calculate SD. We will use the most straightforward one, 'STDEV'. Click on OK at the bottom of the box. A new window should now open up:

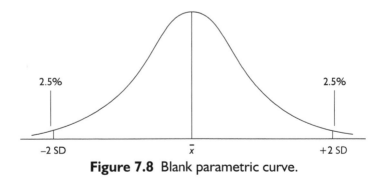

Function Arguments

STDEV

Number1 **D6:D30** = {64;68;71;73;74;76;77;78;78;80;82...

Number2 = number

This is the prompt to either enter the letter and number for the cells you wish to calculate SD for, or to click and drag over the set of numbers in Column A. When you have done this click OK in the function box, and the SD should appear on your spreadsheet.

This gives a SD of 8.48 (it is a standard scientific convention that only the first two decimal places are given).

We now have a value for the mean and standard deviation of population A. What does this tell us?

Take a piece of paper and draw a parametric curve as shown in Figure 7.8.

2.5%   2.5%

−2 SD $\bar{x}$ +2 SD

Figure 7.8 Blank parametric curve.

Write the mean where the letter x is. To the mean, add two times the standard deviation: the mean for population A is 80.75 (i.e. approximately 80); the

SD is 8.5, therefore the upper figure here is 97. Write this in where it says +2SD.

Now repeat this, but subtract two times the SD from the mean and write it in too. Within these two limits approximately 95% of the population lies. These are commonly referred to as confidence limits, because it means we can be confident that this is where most of the population lies. Conversely, only 2.5% of the population exists above the confidence limit and 2.5% below it. This is not just an academic discussion. With a mean and the SD, it is possible to summarise any parametric population, and as will be shown next, this is one of the key concepts behind statistical testing. To be precise, the confidence limits are the mean plus or minus 1.96 times SD, but using the rounded value of 2 is a useful approximation.

Inferential statistics: testing the differences between groups

Figure 7.9 shows two hypothetical populations. These could illustrate two groups of surgical patients. Group A had a standard form of post-operative analgesia, and group B had a new experimental one.

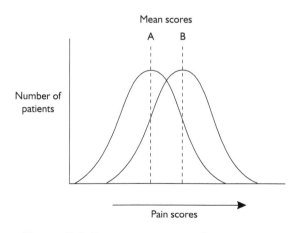

Figure 7.9 First comparison of pain scores.

The figure summarises the pain scores for the two groups. Look at the graph; is it possible to distinguish between the two populations? Do they look significantly different?

Inspection would seem to suggest that if a patient was in group A, they were more likely to have a lower pain score than if they were in group B. There is however, a lot of overlap, so there are a lot of people for whom it does not matter which group they were in – they had similar pain scores. In statistical terms, it is unlikely that they would have a significantly different pain score, regardless of which group they were in. In layman's terms, although it looks as though group A had a lower set of scores, the chart alone cannot show whether the groups were really different.

Now look at the populations in Figure 7.10. This is a similar picture, but this time there is very little overlap between the two groups. Still using the pain scenario outlined above, it looks as if almost everyone within group B has a higher pain score, with very little overlap between the two. This suggests that there is a real difference between the groups, and you may consider that, given the choice, it would be a good idea to sign up to group A.

What these examples show is that when comparing two populations, it is necessary to compare not only measures of central tendency (means, medians and modes), but also the spread of the populations (standard deviations). The branch of statistics which explores these connections between groups is termed inferential statistics.

The classic inferential test to compare two populations is Student's *t*-test. This is only applicable if a population is parametric. A *t*-test compares the two populations and determines whether they can be seen to be statistically sepa-

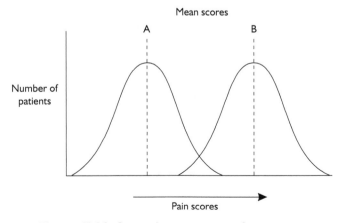

Figure 7.10 Second comparison of pain scores.

rated. It looks at the mean and the spread of the population and compares these to a completely random population.

Examples of unpaired tests could include:

- Using a quantitative questionnaire to score differences in stress between men and women.
- Comparing percentage marks for a group of students taught using a distance learning package with a group using conventional methods.
- Number of days survival of patients following myocardial infarction between those treated with thrombolysis and rescue angioplasty.

Not all sets of data can be assessed this way. Firstly, the independent variable should be interval level (although ordinal data such as those obtained from Likert scales are frequently used), and both populations should be parametric. Lastly, the populations should have similar variance, which really means that the populations should look fairly similar and have similar spreads (as in the examples above).

t-tests can also be paired or unpaired. Unpaired tests explore populations in which the individuals cannot be identified. Paired tests explore the population where the same individuals are measured twice. Paired tests are more powerful, meaning that they have a greater ability to identify differences between groups. Now do Excel exercise 7.

Excel exercise 7

This is the most complex use of Excel to be used in this book. Make sure that you have mastered the previous examples. As before, click on the cell where you would like to the result of the *t*-test to appear.

Max	96	99
Min	64	67
Average	80.75	84.05
Median	81	85.5
Mode	78	81
Sdev	8.48451	8.450942
t test		

Now, in the same way that you looked for the STDEV function in the Auto sum dialogue box, go into More Functions and find TTEST. Click on this in the 'Select a function' box:

Insert Function

Search for a function:

| TTEST | Go |

Or select a category: Recommended

Select a function:

> T
> **TTEST**
> LINEST
> SINH
> TINV

You will now be asked to enter two arrays of data. Click and drag over data set A and its location should appear in the first array box.

Repeat for the second array. Both sets of data have now been entered (the cell numbers will vary according to where you put your original data). There are two final dialogue boxes:

Function Arguments

TTEST

Array1	D6:D25	= {64;68;71;73;74;76;77;78;78;80;...
Array2	E6:E25	= {67;71;74;76;77;79;81;81;83;85;86;
Tails	2	= 2
Type	2	= 2

= 0.225376192

Returns the probability associated with a Student's t-Test.

Type is the kind of t-test: paired = 1, two-sample equal variance (homoscedastic) = 2, two-sample unequal variance = 3.

Formula result = 0.225376192

Help on this function   OK   Cancel

We will assume that there are two tails to this test (this means it is possible for one group to be higher *or* lower than the other) and it is a type two test we want, where the variances for the two groups are similar (as we know that the related statistics, the standard deviations, are similar). Then click OK. The result for the *t*-test should appear like this:

Max	96	99
Min	64	67
Average	80.75	84.05
Median	81	85.5
Mode	78	81
Sdev	8.484506002	7.05279
t test	0.225376192	

Just before we interpret the *t*-test, there is one final point to consider.

Statistical significance

When we inspected the charts comparing pain relief, we found that it was not possible to say that one set of data was absolutely different from the other. If pressed, it might be possible to say that in the second example, one was *very probably* different from the other. The same is true when we run inferential statistics such as a *t*-test. The test will not say that '*set A is definitely different from set B*'; instead it gives a probability, also known as a *p* value.

The smaller the *p* value, the more likely it is that two sets of data are different. Scientists use a *p* value of 0.05 as the cut-off. If a *p* value is 0.05, it means that in 5% (this is another way of writing 0.05) of the cases, the test may get it wrong, but the other 95% of the times the test is run, it has picked up a real difference between groups.

The Excel example which we ran gave a *p* value of 0.22. This is much larger than 0.05, so although the measures of central tendency are all lower for set A, the two sets of data are not statistically different at all! This means that if these data were the result of an experiment, the researchers would have to conclude that there was no real difference between the two treatments and the two drugs were similarly effective. Incidentally, although the cut-off point of 0.05 is universally used, it is actually only a convention. It was introduced by a statistician called Ronald Fisher in the 1920s, and since then has been widely adopted. As Field (2009) has pointed out, if Fisher had woken up one day with a '0.10' feeling, the whole course of science might have been different!

Other tests

t-tests only work with two groups. If there are more than two samples then One Way Analysis of Variance (usually shortened to ANOVA) may be suitable. This test assumes that all groups are equal and drawn from the same population. As with *t*-tests, the independent or grouping variable is nominal but must have more than two levels: for example, gender has two levels (so would require a *t*-test), whereas ethnicity has many levels, so if it were desirable to see if there were differences between groups in a survey, ANOVA would be used. The output is similar, again providing *p* numbers to distinguish between groups.

Non-parametric tests

Fisher was a very busy man, and in addition to determining the significance level, he invented ANOVA and also an entirely new field of inferential statistics: the use of *non-parametric* techniques. As the name suggests, these are used where a population does not have not the classic bell-shaped curve.

These tests make fewer assumptions and are generally held to be less powerful, but they are very valuable, particularly in small research projects.

As before, the first step in data analysis would be consideration of the nature of the population. If it cannot be confirmed that the population is at least approximately parametric, then non-parametric techniques are used. If there are two independent groups, then the Mann–Whitney *U* test would be used, while if there are more than two independent groups, then the Kruskal–Wallis test would be used. These techniques work in a different way from the parametric tests. Rather than comparing means and distribution, the scores are put into ranks. The analysis then compares the ranks. However, the outcome is very similar: a probability is produced and, as before, if the result is smaller than 0.05 then the test groups are statistically different. Figure 7.11 shows a flow chart of the commonly used statistical tests.

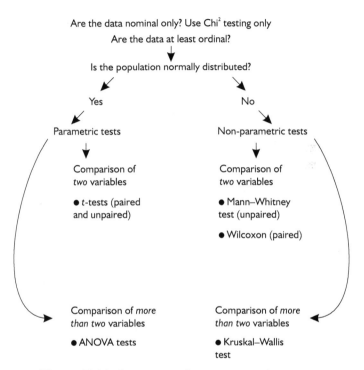

Figure 7.11 Summary of quantitative data tests.

Nominal data testing – the Chi square test

This is the final test to be considered. The preceding discussion has focused on data which are at least ordinal, and ideally would be interval. However, in health research, quite commonly the outcomes are categorical, for example alive or dead, pregnant or not.

If the outcome of a piece of research is categorical and there are two groups involved, then the suitable technique to distinguish between groups is the Chi (pronounced 'ki', to rhyme with 'pie') square test. An example from Argyrous (2005) is shown below:

Place of residence	Low income	High income
Rural	205	118
Urban	167	230

The question here is whether there is a link between place of residence and income. For example, it might be thought that poor people tend to live in inner city areas and the well off in large villas in the country. Is this what is represented here? This sort of table is termed a cross-tabulation and summarises the data clearly. The Chi square test assumes that the two headings (place and income) are not related, i.e. that the variables are independent. As usual it is always a good idea to look at the descriptive data. If these are summarised as percentages, the data appear as:

Place of residence	Low income	High income
Rural	55%	34%
Urban	45%	66%

Inspection shows that those on low incomes actually seem to be over-represented in the rural environment (55%) rather than the urban (45%). If the same pattern exists for the high income group then there is probably no difference between the high- and low-income groups, or income is independent of residence. But if (for example) a greater number of high-income people live in urban areas, this may show that residence is related to income, so income is not independent of residence. Inspection seems to show that there are fewer people from the high-income bracket in the rural environment (34%) rather than urban (66%). The groups therefore seem to be behaving differently, but is this difference statistically significant? Running a Chi square test on this set of data gives a p value of < 0.001. This means less than 1 in 1,000. Clearly this is much smaller than 0.05, so the answer is that these populations really are different: the low-income families are really more likely to live in the rural environment and the high-income ones in urban areas (and vice versa).

This is rather a brief discussion of the use of categorical data, but there is a reason for this. In this example the terms 'low and 'high' income are not defined. With more detailed data, for example income considered in annual bands such as £0–£5,000, £5,000–£10,000 etc., it is possible to be more detailed in the analyses. These data are now interval level, and so (for example) could produce all the descriptive data already discussed and could be distinguished by either a *t*-test or a Mann–Whitney test, depending on the distribution of the population.

As a general rule, it is recommended that when constructing questionnaires you should aim for the highest form of data that can be used, as this will allow the most detailed analysis. Now do Excel exercise 8.

Excel exercise 8: coding ordinal data

Likert scales and other types of ordinal data have been mentioned already. You may remember that an example of one Likert item was given at the beginning of Chapter 5:

	Strongly disagree	Disagree	Neutral	Agree	Strongly agree
I understand a lot about quantitative research					

This was given to a group of 22 third-year midwifery students, who were asked to tick the box which best represented their opinion. The data were distributed as follows:

Student	Strongly disagree	Disagree	Neutral	Agree	Strongly agree
A	✓				
B			✓		
C	✓				
D	✓				
E				✓	
F			✓		
G		✓			
H			✓		
I	✓				
J		✓			

K				✓	
L					✓
M		✓			
N		✓			
O			✓		
P			✓		
Q		✓			
R				✓	
S		✓			
T	✓				
U		✓			
V				✓	

In order to enter them into Excel, these need to be coded. There are a number of different ways this can be done. The statement used is a positive one, so the most intuitive and straightforward way to enter these data is to assign codes as follows:

Statement: 'I understand a lot about quantitative research'. Codes:

- Strongly disagree = 1
- Disagree = 2
- Neutral = 3
- Agree = 4
- Strongly agree = 5

This way, the most positive response gets the highest positive score. Note that if the statement is a negative one, this order may be reversed as follows,

Statement: 'I understand very little about quantitative research'. Codes would be:

- Strongly disagree = 5
- Disagree = 4

- Neutral = 3
- Agree = 2
- Strongly agree = 1

This makes sense, and again is the most intuitive way to code the data. The student who strongly disagrees that they understand little about research, is really stating that they feel they know a lot about research, so in this case a high score should arguably be given. This discussion may seem a little obscure, but if a number of Likert items are used to make a Likert scale, and if half of these are positively orientated (I understand a lot...) and half are negatively orientated (I understand very little about...), then it is important to score the items in this way. This allows the researcher to summate, or add together the scores, in a meaningful way, to give an overall score which represents the data set.

Code the data and enter them into Excel as follows – this should be familiar territory by now. The first five pieces of data have been entered:

Score
1
3
1
1
4

When you have entered the data, you can calculate the mean and median scores as before.

Interpretation

The interpretation of the numbers is based on a minimum possible score of one and a maximum possible score of five. Therefore if the scores were spread evenly across all the five values, a mean score of 3 would indicate an overall neutral point; so if the measures of central tendency which you use fall below this, the respondents are giving a relatively low score (i.e. they are, as a cohort, reporting a lack of confidence), and if they rise above this, they are giving a high relatively score (i.e. they are, as a cohort, reporting that they feel confident).

As before, a chart is a good concise way to show data, and quite reasonable bar charts can be generated in Excel, but they do require a little manipulation. First of all, produce a summary of the data as shown below, and highlight the boxes:

Strongly disagree	5
Disagree	7
Neutral	5
Agree	4
Strongly agree	1

Then click on the Insert tab, and select the Column chart option:

Click on the first option (Clustered column), and a very acceptable bar chart appears:

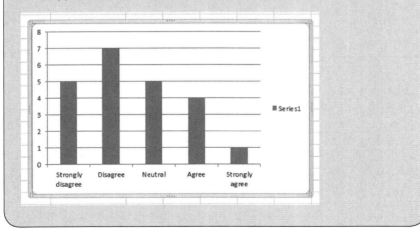

This can actually be edited further by double-clicking on the chart. Although not as flexible as SPSS, this may be entirely adequate for writing up a report or modest research project, and as can be seen, it is very easy to do.

Finally, generating means from ordinal data such as these is not technically correct (or at least is slightly suspect), because it more or less assumes that the data are scaled or interval level, i.e. that the difference between each increment is the same. However, most researchers and analysts do this. If you are not convinced, and if the data look highly skewed, then it might be best to opt for the median value(s), which no-one can argue with.

An introduction to statistical relationships

The statistical techniques explored so far have focused on finding out whether groups can be demonstrated to be different. This is very important, for example in determining if two groups in an experiment show real changes to client outcomes; this could illustrate the effect of a new drug or any other intervention. It is, however, only a start; this final section of the chapter can be viewed as a further 'taster', of what statistics can do. Rather than look for differences, statistics can be used to identify relationships (Sapsford, 2007) between variables, which is also termed modelling. This branch of enquiry can give more insight into the relationship between data sets.

Correlations

The most basic technique, but also one of the most important, is to look for correlations between variables. Figure 7.12 (overleaf) uses another type of chart, a scatter plot, to show the relationship between pain and anxiety in a set of post-operative patients.

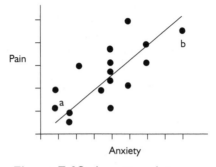

Figure 7.12 A scatter plot.

It can be seen here that as anxiety score increases, the pain score also increases. For example patient 'a' has an anxiety score of 1 and a pain score of 1 also. Patient 'b' is less fortunate: he or she has an anxiety score of 8 and also a pain score of between 4 and 5. This is an example of a positive correlation: as one score increases, the other also increases. It is not a perfect relationship. The drawn line shows the direction of the correlation, but not all data lie on the line. To explore these further, as with techniques for exploring differences between data sets, it is necessary to determine whether the data are parametrically or non-parametrically distributed. If the distribution can be shown to be parametrically distributed, then Pearson's Correlation can be used.

Running Pearson's Correlation gives two statistics. The first of these is the correlation statistic, which is a value between -1 and 1. Since we can be sure that this is a positive relationship, in this case the number for these data will be between 0 and 1. A score of 1 is a perfect correlation, in which case all the data would appear on the drawn line. A score of 0 would mean that there was no relationship at all and the data would be scattered across the plot without a pattern. The other statistic is the level of probability. This has been discussed before, and the same cut-off value of 0.05 is used here. Microsoft Excel does not analyse for correlations, so a more sophisticated statistical package such as SPSS would be used here.

For these data, the output from SPSS is:

Pearson correlation = 0.85
$p = 0.002$

This shows that there is a strong positive correlation between the two data sets and that it is statistically significant. This means we can be confident in saying that as anxiety score increases, so does the patient's pain. What it *does not do* is show that one causes the other, i.e. we do not know if the pain causes the anxiety, or the anxiety causes the pain (or possibly a mix of the two).

If these were non-parametric data, then correlation would be explored by Spearman's rho. In practice, although slightly less sensitive, the same format of result is given, a *rho* value between –1 and 1 and a *p* value.

Figure 7.13 shows an example of a negative correlation.

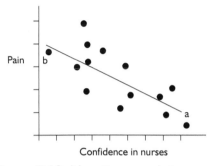

Figure 7.13 Negative correlation.

Here a different picture emerges. Patient 'a' has a high measure of confidence in the nurses (8+) and a low pain score (1), whereas patient 'b' is again unfortunate: he or she has almost no confidence in the nurses (1) and a high pain score (3.5). With a negative correlation, as one index rises, the other falls. This is again summarised with the drawn line. Assuming that these data are not parametrically distributed, Spearman's correlation would be the appropriate choice for exploring the correlation.

For these data, the output from SPSS is:

Spearman's *rho* = –0.5
p = 0.03

The negative value of *rho* shows clearly that this is a negative correlation. It can be seen here that, in addition to it being negative, the correlation is not as large as the previous example. This means that fewer of the data are summarised by the correlation statistic coefficient. This is a moderate correlation, but as the *p* value shows, it is still statistically significant. This means that we can confirm a negative correlation between pain and confidence in the nurses, but as before we cannot comment on causality.

The Pearson correlation statistic and Spearman's rho are both correlation coefficients; they explain the relationship between the two variables. One final refinement is to square these values, to show the amount of data that is explained by the correlation (Field, 2009).

For the first example, which we have identified as having a strong positive correlation, this is 0.85 × 0.85, which equals 0.72, or 72% of the data, i.e. only 28% of the data are not explained by the correlation.

For the second example, a moderate negative correlation, this is –0.5 × –0.5, which equals 0.25, and therefore accounts for only 25% of the data. Note that the negative value becomes lost when the negative correlation is multiplied by itself.

Other modelling techniques

These produce sophisticated models and are not for the faint-hearted. Two techniques will be introduced here. They can be summarised as using predictor variables which explain an outcome variable. An example can be found in Fowler and Norrie (2009), which explored why students might consider leaving their programme of nursing and midwifery studies.

The *outcome variable* was a question: '*Since starting your programme of studies, have you ever thought seriously about resigning or leaving the course?*', which was scored using a Likert scale. A set of predictor variables was given, composed of 27 items which might realistically have an effect on this outcome (for example '*I am finding the volume of work to be too much*'). To explore this, a modelling technique called multiple regression was used, which produced a model showing that eight of these variables were statistically significant, accounting for 33% of the variation within the data. These predictors were then used, with the addition of qualitative data, to produce a tool that is currently being used to support students who are at risk of leaving their studies. This can be seen as an extension of correlational statistics.

One final technique to mention is logistic regression, which measures the chances of an event happening similarly using a set of predictors (see Table 7.2).

Table 7.2 Summary of levels of data in regression analyses.

Technique	Outcome variable	Predictor variables
Multiple regression	At least ordinal	At least ordinal
Logistic regression	Dichotomous nominal	Nominal or ordinal

Although mathematically different from multiple regression, in practice it produces similar types of findings. It is mentioned here because it is used commonly by medical researchers. As you can see from Table 7.2, the outcome variable is dichotomous (two possible choices) and nominal only, e.g. yes or no. This can be useful in medical studies where the outcomes are similarly nominal, e.g. in renal failure (or not) or allergic (or not).

These techniques allow quite sophisticated and robust modelling, but again they cannot show causality. Lastly, beware of statistical techniques like these because they are addictive. You have been warned!

CHAPTER 8

Other strategies and evidence

This chapter pulls together some of the themes which have been explored so far, and will introduce a new one. This is the concept of 'evidence' and the aim is to explore some aspects of what evidence-based practice means for healthcare practitioners. Two important sources of evidence have already been introduced: research findings produced by either qualitative or quantitative inquiry.

These two branches have so far been explored separately. This is a useful strategy when introducing the world of research. However, the split between the two can be overstated. A growing number of researchers are using both branches together to produce findings relevant to practice. A common method is to start out with inductive (i.e. qualitative) methods to identify the phenomena of interest. This is because qualitative work seldom answers questions, but instead produces new theory. In lay terms this means it generates new ideas. This is positive, but the researcher may feel that the work is unfinished, and instead may wish to measure how important, or otherwise, these ideas are in the world of practice. The clue here is in the word 'quantify'; to do this, it is logical to also use deductive (i.e. quantitative) methods (Teddlie and Tashakkori, 2009). Here is an example to work through.

Exercise: tackling the paperwork

Your clinical area has invested £500,000 in an advanced electronic patient data management system. When fully implemented, this will result in a 'paperless' ward environment, which it is hoped will liberate time for medical staff and nurses that can then be spent in delivering patient care.

A lecturer at a local university is keen to participate in the evaluation of this project and will participate in the fieldwork and data analysis, on the understanding that this can be used for a PhD project.

Identify how many research investigations you will include.

A part-time PhD usually lasts five years. Realistically this will result in fieldwork which can span a period of two years, during which the system will come online.

Identify how you would structure the project, bearing in mind that very little has been written about the ways in which health workers use these systems. Include some pre- and post-implementation measures.

Will there be one or more quantitative phases, one or more qualitative phases, or a mix of both?

Discussion

There are many different ways in which this research could have been undertaken. What actually happened was as follows.

A set of interviews was conducted in the clinical area where the system was going to be introduced. The main focus of these was asking the nurses what they wanted from the information system, and what their concerns might be. This therefore was an inductive stage. These findings were compared to a similar clinical area where they previously had used a computerised information system, which had then been discontinued. This allowed an analysis which identified common themes. These themes were then taken and used to construct a 23-item Likert scale, which was used in three clinical areas: two which used conventional manual data recording methods, and one which used a computerised system manufactured by Hewlett-Packard called CareVue 9000. The result of this was that the research identified quite strongly that the computerised system gave consistently higher scores than manual recording, in terms of reliability, time saving and communication. As good PhD students should, these were published shortly after completion of the project as Norrie (2003) and Norrie and Anthony (2004).

In many ways this is a fairly typical PhD project, and does indeed follow the inductive, *then* deductive format identified above. Taken together these findings form a set of evidence which could influence decision making regarding the purchase of such a system.

Case studies

A case study usually investigates a topic within a real-life setting. Therefore there are two conditions. Firstly the physical setting is (usually) clearly stated; for example, the research could take place within a community district, a ward, or an operating department. If required, the case could actually be visited. Secondly, there is a technical or care-related issue which is to be investigated within this setting. In the example given above, it was the introduction of a computerised data system, but the opportunities are endless: the topic could be communication between departments, wound management or attitudes to managing complaints.

In research terms, Yin (2009) described the case study as a strategy for research, rather than a tradition, framework or paradigm. This means that rather than be tied to a particular way of doing the research (for example 'I am a qualitative researcher!'), the investigator can choose whichever methods work best for a particular part of the case study project. This gives a lot of freedom to researchers and is therefore a popular way to proceed. This was confirmed by Bryar (1999) who reviewed a number of nursing case study projects and found that the majority used both qualitative and quantitative investigations within a geographically delineated area.

As well as being attractive, case studies can produce very good quality research. In these, each step taken is demonstrated as being derived from the previous one, and this clear audit trail supports both reliability and validity. The case study has one special attribute: the clear and detailed description of a case can have an impact greater than almost any other form of research report (Gillham, 2000b). Perhaps for these reasons, the case study lends itself well to students undertaking doctorates, where the process of including multiple sources of information and making logical and justifiable steps in the chain of evidence lends itself well to the format of an 80,000 word dissertation (Norrie, 2004).

A clear process is therefore required and a number of decisions have to be made to use a case study well. The researcher should:

1. Define the case, i.e. where the study is taking place and why.
2. Identify the research tools which are best suited to the research questions.
3. Carry out the fieldwork.
4. Analyse the fieldwork.
5. Decide if more fieldwork is needed. If so repeat steps 2–5 again.
6. Integrate the findings through a process of triangulation or mixed methods synthesis.

Participatory action research (PAR): a 'hands on' tradition

This is quite a radical departure from the preceding ones. It has been introduced earlier under qualitative methods, but is re-introduced here because it also allows the integration of a number of different types of research investigations.

All the discussions on quantitative methods so far have been based upon the positivist paradigm. This includes, albeit tacitly, the premise that the research is distinct from the research setting. For example, experiments are typically designed outside of the clinical area, and conducted by researchers who actually make a point of blinding the practitioners involved as to the nature of the experimental interventions they administer, in order to minimise the introduction of bias. The unwritten expectation is that research is done by 'others'; experts from outside the clinical area who can make dispassionate observations and analyses. The extreme case of this would be the Multi-Centre Randomised Controlled Trial, where the researcher may be in a different country from where some (or all) of the fieldwork takes place.

As has been discussed, PAR is a response to this divorcing of research from the clinical area (McNiff and Whitehead, 2006). It is emancipatory, that is, it frees clinical staff to set their own research agendas and to use their knowledge in advancing the research (Morton-Cooper, 2000). They are then no longer subjects of the research: they become the investigators! It is easy to see why nurses, midwives and other practitioners could get excited about PAR; for once, they can become the key players and are not reliant upon 'expert' researchers.

According to Denscombe (2007), action research has four main defining characteristics.

1. It is practical: it is aimed at dealing with real-world issues within clinical settings. The research is undertaken as part of practice, and is not distinct from it. The researchers are partners in the clinical area where care takes place.
2. It involves change: the practitioners are required to focus on their own practice as they engage in that practice. As with case studies, many different methods can be included, as long as they are a good fit for the research needs.
3. It is a cyclical process. The research includes a feedback loop. After (1) reflection on practice, (2) planning of change, (3) acting upon the plan comes (4) observation, before the team decides that the cycle is either complete (their goal has been achieved) or another turn of the cycle is required (their goal has not been achieved).

4. It is participative. Practitioners are the crucial people in the research process. Partnership is therefore a key process in action research.

This is a radical revision of the relationship between researchers and subjects. Like case studies, it encourages the use of a variety of research methods including:

- Reflective tools
- Audit studies
- Focus groups
- Patient feedback surveys

It is included in this section because at the planning stage a number of options become available. In the words of Gilbert and Sullivan in the comic opera *The Mikado*, 'let the punishment fit the crime'. Translated to the world of research, this means that the research questions should dictate the methods to be employed, and as with case studies these can be wide-ranging. This perspective is close to the case study outlook and indeed the action researcher might go further, using not only what may be termed 'accepted' research methods, such as interviews and surveys, but more borderline ones too, for example clinical audit and client satisfaction surveys. This is particularly true where rapid appraisal of the issues is required. Murray and Graham (1995) cite the case of rapid appraisal of health needs of a group of residents in Scotland; the project combined document searches, new fieldwork using qualitative methods, hospital records and a postal survey. This collection would not look out of place in a case study approach, and indeed Denscombe (2007) links action research with case studies in terms of their reliability and validity. The differences are clear, however; with PAR it is the participants within the clinical area who undertake the research and the emphasis is on change, action and evaluation the results of the action.

Bringing sets of data together

Whichever way the project is run, the output remains a number of sets of data. At some point, these have to be brought together to produce a set of findings which will summarise the project and produce findings which can be put into practice. What options are available?

Triangulation

Until recently the most frequently cited way to bring different sets of findings together was through a process called triangulation, publicised by Denzin and Lincoln (2000). This is a technical term used in surveying and navigation. Its principle is illustrated in Figure 8.1. On a flat surface, if two bearings are known then the position of a point can be identified. In this case, X really does mark the spot.

The inference here is that where the findings from the two sets of data cross over, the true findings will be found. There is a lot to be said for triangulation, in that it allows very different sets of data to be included in a research project.

Distinctions have been made between many different types of triangulation; for example *within methods triangulation*, where two sets of methodologically similar data such as interviews are brought together, or *between methods triangulation*, where different types of data such as quantitative data from a questionnaire are compared with qualitative data from a focus group.

There are, however, problems with triangulation that have made it less frequently cited. Firstly, it can be expensive. If the first piece of research answered the research question, it then becomes pointless to spend money on further investigations; the message here would be to formulate a sound piece of research in the first place. Different types of research may give completely different types of results; therefore there may not be any common ground at all between them (Sim and Sharp, 1998).

It is now more common (but not necessarily more correct) to talk in terms of *mixed methods*, which are research projects that contain both quantitative and qualitative investigations. O'Cathain *et al.* (2008) identified that 18% of health service research studies could be classified as using mixed methods, there was even evidence that despite being diehard quantitative researchers, medical staff had started using mixed methods because they were believed to attract funding. The main driver for using mixed methods is to make research more comprehensive, with the acknowledgment that healthcare takes place in complex environments and commonly involves disempowered groups. One

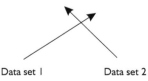

Data set 1   Data set 2

Figure 8.1 Triangulation.

example might be clients with profound learning disabilities, who have difficulties in requesting what they need and whose voices may not be heard in a typical quantitative research structure. Mixed methods therefore are used widely in:

■ Evaluation research, where the quality of a service is explored
■ Surveys, where a large variety of clients are reached
■ Experimental research, where qualitative data are obtained to add context to the main project findings

The 'added value' of these mixed methods is that rather than obtaining one agreed set of findings (as in triangulation), a breadth of findings is found, and it is the differences between data that are at least as valuable as the similarities. This will result in a *meta-inference*. To introduce some of the ways to do this, it will be assumed that there is one research project that has both a quantitative and a qualitative arm. Teddlie and Tashakkori's (2009) classification will be used.

1. **Parallel mixed data analysis**, where the separate data sets are analysed separately. The two sets of data are essentially kept separate during the analysis. The findings relating to the phenomenon under study are combined and linked together at a later stage. However, given that the researchers are likely to be immersed in both aspects of the research project, early findings will shape the analysis of both or either arms.

2. **Sequential mixed data analysis** occurs where the different strands occur in chronological order (e.g. quantitative and *then* qualitative methods), and when the analysis of the first affects the analysis of the second. This is related to *iterative sequential mixed analysis*, which occurs in designs with more than two phases. Iteration means to repeat; in this context it means to return to the analysis on a number of occasions, until a harmonious outcome is produced.

3. **Multilevel mixed data analysis** occurs within research settings such as institutions where there is a hierarchy, for example a ward within a directorate, within a hospital, within an NHS Trust. It occurs when one type of research, for example a set of interviews with patients, is followed by another research method, for example exploring a set of patient satisfaction scores, moving up through the steps of the hierarchy.

4. **Fully integrated mixed data analysis** occurs where a project uses a number of strands that influence each other. Teddlie and Tashakkori (2009) identify that analyses can proceed in parallel, and cross-over of research

types may feature. For example, it may be profitable to quantify qualitative data (how *often* did someone make a comment or statement), and to qualify quantitative data (e.g. produce a description of different subsets within the quantitative data analysis).

With mixed methods analyses, the final analysis integrates and brings the inferences and explanations together in a *meta-inference*. The mechanics of this process are not always made clear. One way of keeping track of findings as they arise which is applicable here, is to write theoretical memoranda as findings and themes emerge (Miles and Huberman, 1994). In practical terms this can be as simple as writing sticky notes of main findings and arranging them on a whiteboard to look for similarities and differences as the data are analysed. Although a very simple technique, it is surprisingly powerful and can help make sense of otherwise very confusing sets of data.

Both triangulation and mixed methods allow research to be developed using a range of investigations. The next two sections illustrate frameworks for including these in a research project which is both rational and cohesive.

Hallmarks of quality in quantitative research

A hallmark is a mark or symbol that guarantees quality. This section will identify research hallmarks, so that the reader can make reasonable decisions about the quality of published research. Traditionally, the quality of research has been discussed under two main headings: Validity and Reliability. These have been applied to both qualitative and quantitative research. They are not necessarily easy qualities to understand, and indeed within the research communities ideas occasionally change when considering the applicability of these to different types of research. To introduce this topic, here is an example which might help illustrate these concepts.

For this example to work, the reader needs to know that, at the time of writing, in Leicester, nurse education takes place at the city campus of De Montfort University. There are a number of charming villages on the outskirts of Leicester which have nothing to do with De Montfort University: Scraptoft and Coalville are two of them.

Is the bus service valid and reliable?

Every morning the number 10 bus arrives outside my house at 08:30 and takes me to the Leicester City Campus of DMU.
It is both reliable and valid.

It arrives on time, but sometimes takes me to Coalville.
It may be reliable but is not valid.

Sometimes it arrives one hour early, but still goes to the campus.
It may be valid, but is not reliable.

Sometimes it arrives at midday and takes me to Scraptoft.
It is neither valid nor reliable!

Translating from this analogy, **validity** can be seen to be an assessment of how well the research addressed the original research question, i.e. '*Did it take you where you wanted to go?*', or in more research-orientated terms, '*Did you answer the question which you set out to answer?*'.

Reliability, in contrast assesses the repeatability or stability of the research. Was the research reliable; *could it be used time after time to produce accurate results?*

Both validity and reliability depend upon each other, which can make discussion of their individual components confusing. For this book it has been decided to discuss validity first, because this is probably where most small-scale researchers are likely to start, by trying to put together a research tool which explores the issues identified in their research question or hypothesis. Once the validity has been addressed, and to some degree assured, it may then be reasonable to start using it in pilot samples, at which point its reliability could realistically be explored. As a final note to this introduction, issues of validity and reliability are seldom resolved. A piece of research is never shown to be either 100% valid or 100% reliable; rather, in a well conducted piece of research these issues are addressed and evidence that they are present is given. Therefore the final judgement of whether validity and reliability have been met is not in the paper: rather, it is in the judgement of the reader.

How to support validity in quantitative research

In the chapter discussing survey literature, a case was made for providing the provenance of questionnaire items; this, it was suggested, supported the validity of the research. It is now time to explore this quality further. In general, it is quite difficult to pin down exactly what validity is, particularly when discussing it in the context of quantitative research. This is because it cannot be directly measured by quantitative or statistical methods (unlike reliability). Instead, it is necessary to review and discuss the research undertaken and look for both its strengths and weaknesses.

Most standard research textbooks supply a glossary of terms. Here is how two popular examples define validity. Polit and Beck (2008, p. 768) define validity as '*the degree to which an instrument measures what it is intended to measure*'. In terms of the earlier example, this is a bus that really *does* take you to the university! This corresponds positively with most other writers, for example, DeVon *et al.* (2007, p. 155) define validity as the '*ability of the instrument to measure the attributes of the construct under study*'. In more everyday language, this equates to 'Did you measure what you set out to measure?', and logically 'Did you answer your research question?'. Thus studies with low validity may well be in-depth and may answer a number of questions – but not necessarily the ones they set out to answer!

Reading about validity also shows that there are a number of components within it. Unfortunately, as Bannigan and Watson (2009) point out, there are rather too many; currently at least 35 different items have been put forward. For the purpose of this book, Polit and Beck's (2008) categories will be used, partly because this book is widely in use in the UK, comes from a highly reputable source, is aimed at researchers working in healthcare, and should be readily available for consultation by students, but mostly because the three main headings are conceptually clear.

A lot of discussion of validity is based around research tools, specifically scales to explore psychometric instruments, such as measures of mood, attitudes and adaptation to illness (DeVon *et al.*, 2007). To discuss it within the context of this book, we will use an example with this in mind. In 2007 Norrie and Dalby used a survey to investigate how student nurses learned, and in particular whether their learning style could be characterised as being 'adult' in nature (andragogic) or 'child' like (pedagogic). A questionnaire was produced and administered to students in years one, two and three of their nursing programmes. This was based upon the work of Malcolm Knowles, an influential

educationalist (Knowles, 1998).The following passages will explore whether this study contains evidence of the different types of validity.

1 Internal validity

Internal validity is described most easily in terms of an experiment. The question which the researcher should ask is 'has the effect that I have discovered come from the independent variable (in experimental terms), or has it been caused by another confounding variable?'. A confounding variable is a variable which has not been recognised and interferes with the results (Pallant, 2010). This is always possible – one candidate might be a Hawthorne effect (discussed in Chapter 5), caused by the subjects being part of a research study itself (Bowling, 2009). A well-conducted experiment will be set up to control this happening by careful sample selection and by randomisation into treatment groups. Surveys are perhaps more susceptible, as no effort is (usually) made to provide a control. Applied to Norrie and Dalby's (2007) research, internal validity is an issue. For example, as the students move from year one through to year three, do they become more exhausted and disillusioned? Are these confounding factors which the research does not take into consideration? Hindsight is always perfect, and in retrospect it might have been better to include other questions to explore (for example) how anxious or fatigued the students felt, to try to find other factors which might, or might not, explain the results.

2 Construct validity

As Polit and Beck (2008, p. 299) point out *'research cannot be undertaken without using constructs'*. A construct is an abstract idea or concept. DeVon *et al.* (2007) state that each item within a research instrument (for example a survey questionnaire) should address an aspect of the construct which is being investigated. In practical terms this means that, when constructing the questionnaire, care must be taken to show that the items included are relevant to the research question, and ideally that they address a specific aspect of it.

An extreme example of bad practice would be the researcher who sits down at his or her desk and draws up a questionnaire using only his or her own knowledge and experience. It is quite possible that the items in the question-

naire are relevant, but there is no proof, and it seems likely that personal bias will compromise the validity of the questionnaire.

By contrast, Norrie and Dalby (2007) based their research on the model (or construct) that they wished to explore. Critical parts of Knowles' work were copied and circulated. Three focus groups were conducted, where sample statements were developed for inclusion in the questionnaire to explore the main elements within Knowles' theory. Therefore a sustained effort was made to support construct validity by a direct link between the theory and the survey.

Another way to support construct validity is to use or amend an existing research tool. There are a number of questionnaires already in existence, such as the Hospital Anxiety and Depression Scale (Zigmond and Snaith, 1983), which as the name suggests explores issues of anxiety and depression and has been used in clients within the hospital and outpatient setting, and the various Short Form questionnaires (e.g. SF-36, SF-12), which are commercially available and have been shown over a long period of time to be valid (and reliable too). These have been discussed in greater detail in Chapter 7.

3 External validity

External validity is a measure of how well the findings relate to the real world. Bowling (2009) relates this to sampling; if the sample is well chosen, then the results can reasonably be expected to be relevant to that defined group of people. For example if conducting research into the effect of tri-cyclic antidepressants such as amitriptyline on chronic pain, the researchers would think carefully about who to include within their study. Ideally the group would be self-identifying, that is people with chronic pain. However, chronic pain is a large and diverse group in itself. Does the research question really identify such a broad group or might it be more specific? Does it include people with neuropathic pain (pain caused by damage to nerves, for which there is a *prima facie* case for effectiveness), or people who have (for example) arthritis, which is both painful and chronic, but is unlikely to respond to these therapies. Again, the correct research question or hypothesis emerges as the critical factor in initiating high-quality research. Another factor is sample size. Small studies are at risk of compromising external validity as small studies involve the risk of sampling bias and type 2 error. This is where an effect exists, but the sample size is too small to demonstrate it. This also raises the issue of how large the sample is, which is discussed in Chapter 5.

In terms of Norrie and Dalby's (2007) paper, the study was interested in how student nurses developed their learning over the three-year period of their nursing studies. Therefore samples were chosen from years one, two and three to follow this progression. A sample size of 321 was used – this was the total number of students who could be persuaded to complete the questionnaire. However, the return rate was only 57%, so bias in response may be present, which could limit the external validity of the work.

Reliability

Bowling (2009, p. 468) defines reliability as '*the extent to which the measure is consistent and minimises random error (its repeatability)*'. Similarly, Polit and Beck (2008, p. 730) define it as '*the degree of consistency or dependability with which an instrument measures the attribute it is designed to measure*'. Bannigan and Watson (2009) use the example of a pole which is claimed to measure one metre in length to illustrate the concept. No matter who approaches the pole, it remains the same length. It is therefore completely reliable. This also addresses Bowling's (2009) second criterion: there can be no random error in the pole itself. In research terms this means that if the research were repeated it would provide (roughly) the same results, no matter who undertook it. For example, if we undertook a survey of how much readers of this book understood the world of research on the Monday (on a scale from 0 to 10), and then repeated it on the Tuesday, assuming that they had not read the whole book in between (or possibly even if they had!) the results would be expected to be similar, if not exactly the same. If this was the case, then the survey could be described as reliable. Note that the second use of the survey is very unlikely to produce identical findings. There is always going to be random variability in the research, but this is acceptable and can be measured and its effect quantified. The beauty of quantitative research is that we can measure reliability in research designs. Here are some ways to do this:

- **Test–retest reliability**: A process for exploring this has been described above. For ordinal and interval data, a coefficient of correlation will be produced. As discussed in Chapter 7, a coefficient of 1.0 would indicate identical data sets, which in reality is unlikely to happen. A coefficient of greater than 0.8 would be considered to be high and would suggest satis-factory reliability (Field, 2009). Similarly for nominal data, a kappa analy-sis would be appropriate. This criterion is also termed *stability* by some authors. Although attractive (it is at least an easy to understand concept), it has a drawback. It is expensive in terms of resources, since it means essen-tially doing the survey twice, so researchers should think twice before including it in a design. One option might be to do a test–retest reliability analysis on two smaller pilot groups, for example.

■ **Inter-rater reliability**: This is very useful where participants are being observed. If a researcher observes someone and records data, they are described as being a 'rater'. For example, hand hygiene is currently (and probably always will be) a big issue in healthcare. If a survey is taken of how long people wash their hands, then inter-rater reliability could be addressed by two researchers simultaneously observing the same group of participants washing their hands. The findings would then be analysed, again using a coefficient of correlation or kappa analysis, as above. At this point, you may think, '*but if observers are watching the same event, then surely they* must *record the same data*'. This is not always the case, how-ever. In the example given it would depend (amongst other things) on how well the research has been designed. For example, exactly when does the hand washing start? Is it:
  – When the participants turn on the tap?
  – When the water touches the hands?
  – When soap is applied?
  – When hand washing movements are first observed?
  – Some other index left up to the choice of the observer?
  Therefore to support reliability a well-formulated research protocol with clear definitions of the included variables is essential.

■ **Internal reliability**: Are the data homogeneous? Homogeneous is a research term which serves to confuse, rather than clarify. It simply means, 'of the same kind', indicating that the data are all showing a similar pic-ture, or are 'pointing in the same direction'. Here is an example which has been used in Chapter 6. If I invite a group of students to my house for dinner, and use a questionnaire to explore a number of factors which con-tribute to the quality of the evening, on a scale from 0–10, I might include the following elements:
  1. The quality of the starter
  2. The selection of wines on offer
  3. The quality of the main course

4. The quality of the dessert
5. The choice of cheeses
6. The conversation and company
7. The background music

If all of the diners really enjoyed every aspect of the evening, they would give high scores for all of these. The responses would be homogeneous. Similarly, if all the diners really hated every aspect of the evening, then this set of responses would again be homogeneous. However, within a set of responses there is usually a mixed pattern. If all, or most, members of the group gave high scores for items one through to five, but low scores for six and seven, then the data remain homogeneous, even though some items attract high scores and some low.

If, however, there was a mix – for example some thought the wine was good but others did not; some thought the conversation was good, others thought it was poor – then for these items the results are *not* internally homogeneous. Rather, they are heterogeneous. In the real world, no set of data is entirely homogeneous. In (very) laypersons' terms the data are usually 'lumpy'.

This can be assessed by a number of techniques, one of which is **alpha analysis**. The most common version of this is Cronbach's alpha, but others are available. This measures the relationship between each item in the questionnaire with every other item. It is expressed in the same way as correlations, e.g. a figure of 1.0 shows a set of data that are completely internally reliable, while a figure of 0 shows a set which is completely unreliable. In most situations, a figure of 0.7, or ideally 0.8 and above, shows that the data have reasonable internal reliability (Field, 2009). This is important, because if this is the case individual questionnaire items can be summated. This means that they can safely be added together and an average generated. This is very helpful for anyone who uses a bank of Likert statements or similar type of scale. If we use the example above, if the Cronbach's alpha value is high, for example 0.82, then to give an overall summary of how well the meal went I can take the summated score for each item and generate the mean, median and mode; if the data are parametrically distributed then a standard deviation becomes valid. This is a sound way to bring together a large amount of data and produce clear overall findings; it would provide a single effective measure of how well the dinner went.

Bringing validity and reliability together

These characteristics do not exist in a vacuum. There is also nothing magical about either. If the research starts off with a clear and precise research question, then to some extent both validity and reliability will be built in. The researcher then needs to think carefully at each step of design, sampling and analysis, referring the process back to the research question. Giving an appropriate rationale for each step of the process tends to support both. Finally, *researchers must always pilot their work*. Please note the emphasis. This means using a small scale trial of the research before devoting time and resources to a full-scale piece of work. Vital feedback from this can then be built into the definitive investigation; not to do so threatens both validity and reliability.

Research and evidence: what are the links and differences?

Throughout this book there has been an emphasis on the application of research findings to influence and underpin clinical practice. Research is a major source of evidence, but there is more to evidence-based practice than finding a promising piece of research and then changing one's own practice. Any positive changes thus produced will be piecemeal and may, quite reasonably, attract opposition. What are the skills necessary to develop evidence-based health-care practice? A good place to start is to consider the types of evidence that are available.

In the 1990s Guyatt, working with Sackett *et al.* produced a very influential hierarchy of evidence, aimed primarily at medical staff (Guyatt *et al.*, 1995). Research was divided into five classes, from Class I, the most robust, through to Class V, the least robust. This hierarchy is still in use, notably in the UK by the National Institute for Health and Care Excellence, amongst others, and is summarised in Figure 8.2.

Class I is the strongest type of evidence and is composed of systematic reviews of a number of Randomised Controlled Trials (RCTs). A systematic review uses explicit and rigorous methods to critically appraise and bring together findings from a number of studies (Mulrow and Cook, 1998). They should be transparent, repeatable, comprehensive and report their methods, so in fact they closely resemble the research process itself. The aim in a systematic review is to compare a range of studies, extract information, bring the findings together and produce robust findings in a meta-analysis. If it is accepted that RCTs are a particularly robust form of evidence, then it is clear that a review composed of RCTs will, in effect, result in a set of findings which is larger than the contributing studies – you may remember that in the world of quantitative research bigger really is better!

Systematic reviews are a large topic in themselves, and will not be explored further in this book. There is some good information on how to construct systematic reviews available from the Centre for Reviews and Dissemination (CRD) at York University, UK (http://www.york.ac.uk/inst/crd/funding.htm). Of possibly greater interest is the Cochrane Library (see exercise below).

Class II should be familiar to readers of this book. This contains a single or a few RCTs. Similarly, Class III includes a mix, but these can be described as quasi-experimental studies: those with some, but not all, of the qualities of a true experiment. They commonly lack randomisation between groups of participants. This impairs their ability to identify cause and effect. Class IV moves out of the realm of experiment altogether, and could include surveys, cohort studies, case studies or even action research projects. Finally, Class V contains a mix of other, slightly vague categories; you get the feeling that the authors had rather lost interest here. What is particularly interesting for nurses and midwives is that qualitative research is not included in the hierarchy at all.

Class I: Evidence from at least one systematic review of multiple well-designed Randomised Controlled Trials

Strongest evidence

Class II: Strong evidence from at least one properly designed Randomised Controlled Trial of appropriate size

Class III: Evidence from well-designed trials without randomisation, single group cohorts, time series or matched case control studies

Class IV: Evidence from well-designed non-experimental studies from more than one centre or research group

Class V: Opinions of respected authorities based on clinical evidence or reports of expert committees

Weakest evidence

Figure 8.2 Hierarchy of evidence.

This is not surprising, given that it was developed for medical staff who function largely within the scientific tradition.

Other hierarchies

This classic way of looking at evidence is dominated by medical science, for whom it was developed. As nurses and midwives, we should be aware that it has some weaknesses, the most obvious of which is that there is no place for qualitative research at all (McSherry *et al.*, 2002). As we have seen, qualitative research is based within the interpretivist paradigm, and answers client-focused questions. To address these issues, a different hierarchy has been developed by the Joanna Briggs Institute (JBI). The JBI, although hosted in the University of Adelaide, is an international collective involving over 54 centres and groups, providing evidence from over 90 countries (Joanna Briggs Institute, 2012a). It has been very influential in developing sources of information for healthcare workers to develop their practice. The JBI makes a distinction between effectiveness and economic assessment, which it closely aligns with randomised controlled trials, in levels of hierarchy which are essentially similar to Guyatt and Sackett's hierarchy (above). However, they make a distinction when it comes to assessing evidence for feasibility, appropriateness and meaningfulness (see Table 8.1) (Joanna Briggs Institute, 2012b).

Some explanation may be useful here. Meta-synthesis is a term applied to the qualitative equivalent of meta-analysis. This means that a range of qualitative sources are obtained, and a process of data translation and synthesis

Table 8.1 Simplified JBI levels of evidence.

	Feasibility, appropriateness, meaningfulness
Level 1	Metasynthesis of research with unequivocal synthesised findings
Level 2	Metasynthesis of research with credible synthesised findings
Level 3a	Metasynthesis of text/opinion with credible synthesised findings
Level 3b	One or more single research studies of high quality
Level 4	Expert opinion

– literally producing new findings – takes place. Walsh and Downe (2005) point out that this is still quite a new academic procedure, and that a settled or agreed methodology for meta-synthesis has not yet been developed, so this may include a range of approaches.

The JBI levels are clearly designed to include qualitative research. Level 1, again the strongest form of evidence, specifies a meta-synthesis with unequivocal synthesised findings. This means that, taken together, the findings from the research which has been reviewed produce essentially one set of unified findings. Level 2 substitutes 'unequivocal' with 'credible', this means that although there may be some disagreement between the sources, the main synthesis can be seen as being believable and has truth. Level 3a allows the inclusion of a wider range of sources, including evidence from non-research sources (for example clinical guidelines could be included here), whilst Level 3b allows the inclusion of a single research source, which could be either qualitative or quantitative. Level 4 allows for expert opinion, so this is similar to the Guyatt and Sackett hierarchy.

Cochrane Library

The Library is named after Dr Archie Cochrane, an early pioneer in evidence-based Practice. Of particular interest within the library is the Cochrane Database of Systematic Reviews. This is available from www.thecochranelibrary.com/.

Within the UK it currently appears to be available free of charge for two-page summaries, but in the USA there are reports of limited availability due to charges being imposed. If you have trouble accessing it, use an academic library website, from a local university for example, or from an NHS Trust.

Cochrane Library exercise
Log on to the Cochrane Library website (URL above). Take a look through the 'HIGHLIGHTED NEW AND UPDATED COCHRANE REVIEWS' section on the home page. Scroll through three of the reviews and get a feel for the type of evidence used, the methods and the way that information is provided. Take some time to reflect on whether this format would be helpful to you in developing your practice.

Accessing evidence

One of the problems with trying to access evidence is that there is so much of it! This is an issue that Archie Cochrane identified and was one of the drivers in setting up the Cochrane Library. Approximately 20,000 trials are published each year and around 1,000 articles are added each day to the literature. Fortunately, we also live in an age where we can use technology to address this and simplify our choices, through the use of academic databases. Before discussing finding evidence through a database, it is worthwhile to introduce some terms.

■ **Sensitivity (recall)**
This is a measure of the comprehensiveness of a search method, i.e. its ability to identify all relevant articles on a given topic. Highly sensitive strategies tend to have low levels of precision and vice versa.
    In other words, it may result in large numbers of articles, but not all will be relevant.
■ **Specificity (precision)**
This is a measure of the search strategy's ability to identify articles which deal effectively with the topic, and describes the ability of a search to exclude irrelevant articles. A high-specificity search may result in too few articles, but of these a high number are likely to be relevant.

There are two main types of searches:

■ **Unfiltered databases**
Examples of these include the British Nursing Index (BNI) and the Cumulative Index of Nursing and Allied Health Literature (CINAHL). These are accessible through most UK university libraries. If unsure, ask your local librarian. As the name suggests, the BNI is produced by a group of British Libraries, and CINAHL operates out of California. Taken together, the majority of the English language publications relating to healthcare can be accessed by these through a computer keyboard.
    Using suitable key words, a very quick search can easily be undertaken. To help this process, every year more articles can be accessed as full text. The key words can be referred to as *inclusion* terms; articles which have these terms in their titles or attached key word tabs will be picked up by the search engine. The sensitivity of the search is an issue: amongst the large number of

articles, some and possibly most of them may not be relevant. Boolean operators such as 'AND' are helpful here, as they direct the database to identify articles which include a number of key words. A good tip is to include the term 'AND nurs*' or AND midw*. AND is the Boolean operator, and the use of the truncation symbol (*) means that any term which includes the four letters 'nurs' or 'midw' will be picked up e.g. nurse, nurses, nursing, or midwife, midwives or midwifery etc. Either word on its own is of little use, but when they are incorporated with another search term (e.g. 'Down's Syndrome'), it increases specificity markedly, so that only articles which have a significant nursing or midwifery related content are found. Otherwise the researcher has to wade through highly technical articles on chromosome structure. Even so, the use of inclusion criteria only may result in too many articles. Commonly therefore, it is necessary to start *excluding* some articles, and this could be done according to:

– **Date**: for example to exclude articles older than five or 10 years
– **Language**: typically to include only articles written in English
– **Full text**: if there are really large numbers, then it is possible to be fussy: the searcher can specify only references which include full text, excluding all others.

■ **Filtered databases**

In a filtered database, a number of filters are already in place. The example used here is provided by PubMed, a medical database which is produced by the US National Library of Medicine. As above, it is easy to access through the Internet, and is freely available globally. It can be used similarly to the BNI and CINAHL as an unfiltered database, but in the home page of PubMed, is the heading 'PubMed Tools'. Within this there is a link 'Clinical Queries'. This section has a set of filters built into it, so that any key words that are entered automatically have an extensive set of filters applied to provide results based largely upon randomised clinical trials – very much working within a medical, scientific paradigm.

Using information to make clinical decisions

According to Glasziou *et al.* (2003), the first step in using good-quality information is to set an answerable question. One way to do this is to set a PICO. The letters identify, P for Population (or Patient), I for Intervention, C for Comparator (or Control) and O for Outcome.

PICO Example I

Here is an example: my daughter has a dog bite on her leg. It looks clean and does not require stitches. Should I take her to our General Practitioner for prophylactic antibiotics? Using the PICO format I produce a question:
Should someone who has a dog bite (P) take antibiotics (I) rather than just observe the wound (C) for infection (O)?
In key words this is summarised as:

P   dog bite
I   antibiotics
C   observation
O   infection

Putting these terms into PubMed clinical queries produces a number of results. As of the time of writing (December 2012), there is one direct hit of a small scale study showing no difference between wounds treated with prophylactic antibiotics and those without; but this is quite old, has a limited sample size and uses an antibiotic not currently used in the UK (Elenbaas *et al.*, 1984). Stronger evidence is available on the same page with a direct link to a systematic review from the Cochrane Library entitled 'antibiotic prophylaxis for mammalian bites' (Medeiros and Saconato, 2001).
As discussed earlier, Cochrane Library reviews are as good as it gets in the world of evidence-based medicine, and sit at the top of the quantitative hierarchy of evidence, so within five minutes it is possible to put together a PICO, enter them into a database and, with a little interpretation, get strong evidence for guidance.

What does the evidence show?

Medeiros and Saconato's (2001) review showed that the use of prophylactic antibiotics was associated with a statistically significant reduction in the rate of infection after bites by humans. However, prophylactic antibiotics did not appear to reduce the rate of infection after bites by cats or dogs. Prophylactic antibiotics were associated with a statistically significant reduction in the rate of infection in hand bites.

Given that my daughter was bitten by a dog in her leg, there is no evidence to suggest that prophylactic antibiotics will be helpful, and assuming her tetanus vaccination is up to date I decide to adopt a policy of 'watch and wait'.

Exercise: DIY PICO!

Take five minutes to produce a PICO of your own. This could be about something that has concerned you in practice, but for a change, think about your family and friends. Does your uncle Bill, for example have a cough which won't go away? Does your sister complain of headaches? Are you worried that all this research has made you drink too much alcohol?

Put your PICO in the British Nursing Index (BNI) or a similar database.

Take 10 minutes to look at the results. Decide whether you have been:

Too specific: this is essentially where your search has been too fussy and by including all the terms that you wished it has 'overshot', resulting in very few, and possibly no, hits.

The remedy here is to remove some keywords – are all these terms really necessary? Start to remove some of the less important ones and see if the number of hits increases.

Too sensitive: this is where your search is too broad – you have lots of hits, but it would take too long to look through them.

The remedy here is to start to include some more keywords. Think about how you can narrow your focus. As you add terms, see what it does to the number of hits: they should decrease.

Personal preference will differ, but one way to judge how good you are with your search strategy is to identify how many hits you would be willing or able to sift through on screen over a period of 10 minutes. As a start, aim for a total number of hits no greater than 15.

PICO Example 2

Here is another example of using PICO, with a little more mathematics involved. I am going to travel to a conference on research methods in Singapore. I have a friend who suffered a deep vein thrombosis (DVT) from a similar long-haul flight, and I am wondering if I should purchase some support stockings for the flight. My PICO therefore is:

P   Air travel
I   Stockings
O   Deep vein thrombosis

NB: a comparison was not included, as the comparison was with travellers who did not wear stockings. The greater the number of terms included, the greater the specificity, but the lower the sensitivity. This may be a matter of personal preference, but on the whole it is preferable to have a broader set of sources and then select the study which best meets the clinical query.

As with Example 1, a Cochrane systematic review was found (Clarke *et al.*, 2006), entitled 'Compression for preventing deep-vein thrombosis in airline passengers'. This reviewed 10 randomised trials which compared groups of travellers who wore compression stockings with those who did not. The total number of participants was 2,856.

In these trials 50 travellers on long-haul flights out of a total of 2637 were found to have DVT. Three had worn stockings, 47 had not.

Some mathematics: which group was more at risk?

The risk to a flyer who does not wear compression stockings therefore is 47 divided by 2637, which equals = 0.0178 (or 1.78%).

The risk to a flyer who does wear compression stockings is 3 divided by 2637 = 0.0011 (or 0.11%). There is clearly a reduction between the two groups, but by how much?

Relative Risk = risk of outcome in the stocking group, divided by the risk of outcome in the non-stocking group = 0.0011/0.0178 = 0.062

This tells us how many times more likely it is that an event will occur in the treatment group relative to the control group. A relative risk less than 1 means that the treatment reduced the risk of the outcome. If RR were greater than 1, then we would conclude that the treatment had *increased* the risk of the outcome taking place. Clearly a risk reduction has taken place, showing that wearing compression stockings has had an impact on the occurrence of DVTs.

What else does the mathematics tell us?

If we want to get a measure of whether it is helpful to wear compression stockings in real-life situations, it may be best to work out the Absolute Risk Reduction (ARR), and the Number Needed to Treat (NNT).

As the name suggests, ARR tells us about the absolute difference between the two groups. It is found by subtracting the two rates.

ARR = risk of DVT in the non-stocking wearing group minus the risk of DVT in the stocking wearing group. For this example:

ARR = 0.0178 − 0.0011 = 0.0167

This tells us that wearing compression stockings decreases the chance of DVT for someone undergoing a long-distance flight by 1.67%. The differences between the two groups therefore are relatively small. At this point it might be worth thinking about whether this small change in risk is worth pursuing. Compression stockings, after all, are really not fashionable.

The final way to address this is to look at the Number Needed to Treat.

NNT is useful: it tells us how many people would need to wear stockings in order to prevent one case of DVT. This is worked out by dividing the ARR into 1 (1/ARR). In mathematical terms it is the reciprocal of the ARR.

For this example, 1/ARR = 1/0.0167 = 59.8

The number is always rounded up, as you cannot have 0.8 of a person. This tells us the number of people we need to apply stockings to in order to prevent one case of DVT, i.e. we need to apply stockings to 60 people to be confident that we have reduced the incidence of DVT by one in a population. The Number Needed to Treat tells us not only whether a treatment works, but how well it works. It is useful to healthcare professionals because it gives information on the effort needed to achieve a particular outcome (Talluri, 2005).

What you may have decided by now is that the numbers have limitations. There is a beneficial effect due to wearing compression stockings, but it is small. If you are in a low-risk group, then you may decide that it is not really worth the cost of buying or the rigmarole of applying compression stockings. However, the review is not only about statistics. In the report, some expert opinion is also applied. Clarke *et al.* (2006) also point out that wearing stockings had a significant impact on reducing oedema of the lower legs and that no significant adverse effects of wearing stockings were reported. Therefore if you are in a risk group for DVT, or from previous experience found that flying gave you uncomfortable swollen legs, you may decide that it is worth the cost and trouble to wear stockings (or you may not – this is your choice, but at least you can make an informed choice based upon sound evidence). Now have a look at the exercise on p. 181.

Number needed to harm

The relative risk shows that the new drug (anagrelide) is actually more harmful than the older control (hydroxyurea). The effect is the opposite of the previous example; instead of now calculating the Number Needed to Treat, we now calculate the Number Needed to Harm (NNH). Otherwise the process is identical:

What is the absolute risk?

Absolute risk = 0.1356 – 0.0891= 0.0465

What is the number needed to harm?

NNH is found by dividing the ARR into 1 (1/ARR).

Therefore **NNH** = 1/0.0465 = 21.50

Again the number is rounded up. This means that for every 22 patients who take anagrelide, there will be one who experiences a blood clot, in comparison with the hydroxyurea group.

NB: this was taken to be so strong an effect that the trial was completed early and the recommendation was made that hydroxyurea should be the main treatment for this condition.

Relating evidence to practice

The PICO is nothing if not focused. Indeed, Glasziou and his group intended it as part of the armoury of the busy general medical practitioner in the UK who

A mathematical exercise

Essential thrombocythaemia is a condition where the bone marrow produces too many platelets. Amongst other things, this puts people at risk of clotting and potentially experiencing strokes and heart attacks. An RCT was conducted by Harrison *et al.* (2005) of two medication regimes. One was for hydroxyurea, an established drug that has some rather unpleasant side-effects but definitely reduces platelet counts. The other drug was anagrelide, which had fewer serious side-effects and theoretically might be a preferred option. In a total sample size of 809, the participants were randomised into two groups and treated with the drugs as follows. The total number of blood clots per group was recorded. For this example, we will treat the hydroxyurea group as the control, and compare it with the 'new' drug anagrelide. The data are summarised below:

Drug	Number in group	Number of clots
Hydroxyurea plus aspirin	404	36
Anagrelide plus aspirin	405	55

Work out the risk for each group

Risk for hydroxyurea group =

Risk for anagrelide group =

What is the **Relative risk** for a patient taking anagrelide compared to hydroxyurea? Is this greater than or less than one? What does this tell you?

Relative risk = <u>Risk for anagrelide group</u>
                  Risk for hydroxyurea group

(answers given at the end of the chapter)

is faced with a rapid presentation of patients at surgery and who has approximately two minutes to put a query together and find an answer to it.

The PICO, specifically when it is linked to filtered databases such as PubMed Clinical Enquiry, is perhaps *too* focused. It can be likened to a lighthouse, which sends out a beam of extremely bright light, but surrounding this is a vast shadow. It trades a very high specificity for low sensitivity. In general, for both nurses and midwives it can be suggested that broader, more sensitive searches may work better, reflecting the fact that there are some major differences between the ways in which medicine, nursing and midwifery look at and use evidence. For medical staff, evidence is primarily quantitative in nature and closely linked to large RCTs. It is used to explore the effectiveness of therapies. This is an important goal, but the evidence really only addresses one type of question: 'Does therapy A work better than therapy B?'.

For nurses and midwives we believe that this is too limiting. One significant difference is in the use of qualitative research, which as the earlier chapters of this book have shown, is a major tool for nurses and midwives who wish to develop their practice. Sackett (who coined the phrase 'evidence-based medicine') *et al.* (1996) suggested that the best research evidence should be 'clinically relevant research, often from patient centred clinical research'. The topics chosen for medicine are commonly focused on diagnostic tests and treatments, and may be addressed properly using the first Evidence Hierarchy. Nursing and midwifery are broader and must therefore use a broader range of evidence. Topics chosen for practice development are often situated within the interpretivist paradigm; therefore evidence for these should also be sought within the interpretivist paradigm (Smith *et al.*, 2004): for example 'What are our clients' experiences?' or 'How can we support our women further?'. This means that both qualitative and quantitative research should be used to provide evidence-based nursing practice.

Final exercise: construct your own hierarchy of evidence

In reading this book, you will have learnt about many different ways to do research and to identify evidence. This final exercise is one that only you can do. On a separate piece of paper, sketch out all the different types of research and evidence that you have read about.

Now give them a score, starting with the strongest. Identify the types of research which you would essentially be confident to base your own practice upon most of the time. You could do this by giving a percentage score to each, where:

- ■ 100% would be types of research or evidence that you would always feel confident in using to make practice decisions
- ■ 50% would be where you might be confident (roughly) half the time in using it to make practice decisions
- ■ 10% would be evidence that you would perhaps not use on its own, but might have some value in a larger context

As you can see, it is not possible to be too categorical about attaching these scores, so do it quickly, without too much internal debate.

Use these weightings to construct your own hierarchy, as shown in Figure 8.2.

Finally, compare the two. You may now be able to make decisions about your own evidence outlook. Are you largely an interpretivist, with a leaning towards qualitative data sources, or are you a positivist, more confident in scientific enquiry? Are you somewhere in between? Are you just confused? One possible solution is the use of a pragmatist paradigm, as suggested by Teddlie and Tashakkori (2009), when discussing mixed methods research. To be pragmatic means to focus on practical rather than theoretical considerations, and it could be argued that this is congruent with practice generally, as both nurses and midwives are grounded in practice rather than theory (you are welcome to disagree with this statement – it is a personal opinion). The logical extension of this perspective would be to commend mixed methods to researchers, where the research question dictates the methods, rather than belonging to a 'qualitative' or 'quantitative' camp.

Whichever you choose, you will have clarified something important for your future practice.

Within the discussion regarding case studies and participatory action research, it was shown that the researcher had freedom to choose which research methods best answered the research questions. Similarly when developing a nursing or midwifery evidence base, we have to ask what are the areas of practice we wish to develop, within which paradigm do they exist and, following this, identify where we would look for the best evidence.

Answers for hydroxyurea/anagrelide exercise

Risk for hydroxyurea group = 36/404= 0.0891 (8.9%)

Risk for anagrelide group = 55/405= 0.1356 (13.56%)

Relative risk = 0.1356/0.0891= 1.5219. This value is greater than one, meaning that the people in the anagrelide group were more likely to have a blood clot than those in the hydroxyurea group.

CHAPTER 9

How to do research in the real world

Preparing a bid for research grants

As you read this, you might reasonably think that this chapter is of little inter-est to you, in that preparing a bid is not something you have considered or think a likely activity in the near future, being (as you probably are) engaged in developing your practice and focused on the delivery of high-quality care for patients, clients, families, mothers and their babies. However, integral to the development of practice and delivery of high-quality care is the notion that excellence in care depends on both research and development (R&D). Without R&D, healthcare practitioners would not be able to underpin practice.

The Royal College of Nursing (RCN) has suggested that the potential for nurses to deliver excellence in care has been thwarted by limited research and development capacity and capability in nursing throughout the UK, and a nursing culture that does not universally value research and development (Royal College of Nursing, 2003). The Royal College of Midwives (RCM) holds a similar view when stating that midwives are increasingly interested in making changes to their practice and exploring the effect of these changes. However, the formal process of research training to enable them to develop the necessary skills in this area often appears daunting (Crozier, 2009). We include both midwives and nurses when suggesting that a skills deficit exists in writing research bids and proposals, with the consequence that research projects are often led by the medical profession and other healthcare profes-sionals well versed in carrying out research. Nurses and midwives, more often than not, are involved in recruiting participants into studies, collecting data, and sometimes, but not always, analysing data, but they are not necessarily determining the research focus, leading the project or 'owning the research'. This chapter aims to address this skills deficit in providing the underpinning knowledge for preparing a bid and writing a research proposal. However, as with everything in this book, we are reliant on you to put theory into practice – i.e. *have a go for yourself.* Hence this chapter encourages and promotes a 'how to do it' approach.

The first steps you will need to undertake involve gaining an insight into what funding sources are available to you. This is a fairly simply task, and can usually be undertaken from a desk position, i.e. using your Internet access. However, it does require you to understand where your research is located from a discipline or subject point of view. What we mean here is what theoretical framework underpins where you are coming from. For example, my (SD) recent research work involves consideration of volunteerism and volunteers within the caring professions. I successfully applied for funding from Macmillan Cancer Care, because, as you may know, this organisation provides support to patients and families suffering with cancer, and draws extensively on a community of volunteers to realise the organisation's aims and objectives. The research project was of interest to Macmillan Cancer Care in terms of its potential to impact positively on the work they undertake, and Macmillan subsequently agreed to fund the project.

Once you have an idea of the funding sources of relevance to your research you will need to look in more detail at the particular requirements of those funding bodies, because requirements and stipulations often exist. For example, funders might organise their funding arrangements within streams, such as a technology stream or an education stream. Often funders will 'put out' a specific call for applications based on a perceived need, which may be prompted by a recent government report or a significant health development that requires sustained and systematic investigation. Often experienced researchers will be aware that these calls are coming and will have a research bid prepared well in advance, so you need to be aware of the opposition.

It is imperative that you have a good knowledge of your organisation's R&D arrangements in order that you can maximise your own time and effort, avoid duplication of effort, and harness the expertise available in your workplace, be it the NHS, the voluntary sector, private sector or university. Finally, it is well worth accessing information from funding bodies regarding what makes for a successful application to that particular funder. Often previously funded projects are made available to view on the website, and it is a good idea to read through these with a critical eye, noting how were they written, how much detail was included, and where the emphasis was placed. To get a feel for some of this topic, take a look at the calls for bids from the National Institute of Health Research (http://www.nihr.ac.uk/proposals/Pages/default.aspx).

Once you have undertaken some preliminary thinking, reading and perusing of funding bodies' websites, the next step is to prepare to write a research bid. Clear and concise guidance is best, so some suggestions are presented here. The following logical steps are those we consider essential when considering preparation of a research bid for the first time:

1. **Clarity**. It is important to avoid overusing technical jargon in an effort to try to make your research bid sound 'academic'. What is far more important is to show why and how this research is worthy of funding, why this particular funding body is the right one for this research, and what difference or impact this funding will make on the ability of this research to be carried out. Funding bodies will want to see clarity of thought and a mindful approach to these questions within the research bid.
2. **Review the literature**. Recognise and cite the work of others, while considering and identifying how your research is different and adds to what is known about the topic. Funders will need to be assured that you are not duplicating research effort, as after all we are talking about public money here.
3. **Plan your approach**. How do you intend to carry out your work, i.e. methods and scheme of intended work? In simple terms, what you intend to do, how you intend to do it, how long it will take, and who will be affected by your actions (i.e. ethical issues). This will form the basis of your research proposal (see next section).
4. **Consider the intended outcomes**. What will the impact of this research be, should you be successful? A good approach here is to imagine that you are successful, i.e. suspend all knowledge of how many bids are successfully funded or not, depending on the way you look at it, and simply imagine that your research project *has been* funded. Now, what do you expect the impact will be? Who are you going to talk to about your research and how are you going to do this, i.e. what are your plans for dissemination?
5. **Cost the project**. Funders will need to know, and indeed expect you to be able to tell them, the answer to the million dollar (or pounds and pence rather) question, i.e. what this research will cost, how much you are asking for, and why? This will need to be an extremely well thought out and detailed section. Any request for funding obviously will be open to serious scrutiny. You must include all the details the funder asks you for. It might

be the case that a funding body requires a pre-bid proposal that requires less detail than a full proposal. However, in the spirit of being positive, you will need to consider exactly how much money you need in order to undertake the excellent research project you have described, in readiness for your success. This means you must have considered everything you will need, be it funding for a research assistant, yourself, equipment, travel, transcription, and dissemination, including attendance at relevant conferences. It is worth noting here that funding bodies may restrict what you can apply for in terms of available funds. Therefore, part of preparing for a bid is to check the funding body's website as part of your mindful approach to your research project. If you are not used to providing a budget (plus individual costings), it might be a good idea to include someone in your research team who is: for example a business manager or accountant.

6. **Collaboration and support**. Finally, garner all the support you can. If you are inexperienced and this is your first bid for research monies, ask others to help you. Quite often experienced researchers will be delighted to be added to your bid. They may or may not want to be fully funded for their time. What is important to you is what they can bring to the bid, how they can increase your chances of success, and what you can learn from them. (Adapted from Bournemouth University, 2013).

Writing a research proposal

A research proposal is a summary, brief or otherwise, of how you would actually construct and undertake a research project. As such, it is wise to minimise the theory that underpins the proposal, whilst being more focused on the practicalities of undertaking it; as is said in the newspaper industry, make sure that the proposal addresses: Who, What, Where, When and Why – the essentials of a story. This means that although it is satisfying to have mastered the concepts that underpin the research process, the proposal is probably not the place to exhibit your knowledge – keep it practical! This section will draw on content that has already been introduced, but the context is different. To signpost sections which cover content in greater detail, look out for the '*Key content*' labels, which will identify chapters that might be useful to for you to re-visit.

Logical ordering is important. Research proposals are usually reviewed by non-academics and so need to be accessible. This is not the same as dumbing down; rather, it is necessary for the applicant to write with simplicity and clarity. The proposal needs a clear narrative, i.e. a story. Start with the broadest category first. A very useful concept to help with this is provided by Phillips and Pugh (2005). They suggest that in academic writing it is a good idea to move from background to focal theory. This means that more general, broad topics (background) are discussed first and then the narrative moves on to discuss more applied ones (focal).

Think of this process as a funnel (Figure 9.1). Each step in the proposal should move the reader forward; it should form a logical narrative and move from general to more focused topics. Transferred into a research proposal context, the literature review should inform the research question; the research question should inform the methodology; the methodology informs the methods chosen; and so on. It also means that repetition should be minimised, if not avoided altogether. This funnel approach seems simplistic at first, but it is surprisingly powerful – it tells you what to do and when to do it; you may find it useful in future study as well.

Background

Focal

Figure 9.1

Writing a proposal Part 1: literature review

As we have seen earlier, good quality research builds upon the findings of earlier workers; this is indeed part of the scientific method. Therefore a sound starting point is to explore what previous researchers have found by conducting a literature review. The first step of this is to conduct a literature review. (*Key content* → *Chapter 8*). A set of key words are entered into a high-quality academic database such as CINAHL or BNI. A top tip is to start out with relatively few key words to produce a highly sensitive search, and then to add in more keywords, one at a time, to make it more focussed. This makes the search more specific. As the proposal may be used to bid for money, or may end up being reviewed by an NHS Research Ethical Committee, this needs to be done to a high standard, and clearly more casual sources such as Wikipedia or Google should not be mentioned here (even if they were used!).

The number of sources required should be considered. This is a justification for the research proposal and not an independent literature review, so clearly this is a discussion in the 'how long is a piece of string?' category. However, it could be suggested that for a proposal to undertake research within the NHS for a Masters or higher degree, the literature review in the proposal should not be longer than two sides of A4 paper, and could contain reference to 5–10 key sources. Again, although quality is important, the narrative is probably more relevant here, as the evidence leads on to the next section: the production of the research question. Therefore, discussions of quality such as data extraction may well not be required, but the forward direction of the research is. For example, it might be best to review the evidence in chronological order, effectively building on what previous workers did up until the present, thereby acting as a springboard for *your* research.

Writing a proposal Part 2: Identification of the research question/hypothesis

This section is really central to any proposal. A well-written research question, or hypothesis, gives guidance and underpins the project (*Key content* → *Chapter 6*). Research questions tend to be open-ended and are used for inductive enquiry. These tend to be projects which explore new territory. An example might be useful here. One of the authors of this book (PN) bid for a research budget to explore the ideal qualities of future cohorts of student nurses, who would be starting the all-graduate intakes from 2012/13. The initial review of literature was rather disappointing and the relevant variables were not clear, so it was decided to approach this with an open-ended research question:

How can we select the right students to undertake all-graduate nursing programmes?

This is clearly very a very broad question; although it allows a good degree of freedom for the research team, the project still needs more guidance. To do this it was then broken down into three main aims:

1. *To determine from a range of perspectives key characteristics required by students applying for entry to nursing in the new all-degree curriculum*
2. *To establish a profile of the ideal characteristics required for students applying for entry to the new all-degree curriculum*
3. *To search for innovative practice to assist identification of high quality students in the new all-degree curriculum*

Taken together this provided suitable guidance for the research project. This is a common mode of preparing research questions, suitable for bidding for small scale projects, Masters and even PhD projects. The other option here is to set a hypothesis (*Key content* → *Chapter 5*). A hypothesis is a statement of the relationship between variables. In this book it has been suggested that the researcher utilise the structure of a PICO (Glasziou *et al.*, 2003) – that is, the hypothesis identifies the Participants, Intervention, Comparison and Outcomes to be studied. In research proposals there may be a number of hypotheses proposed or, as with the example given above, one main hypothesis, with a number of subsidiary aims.

Note that open-ended research questions work well with qualitative and survey projects. If you are going to use an experiment, a hypothesis is required.

Writing a proposal Part 3: Selection and rationale for research methodology

In a research proposal limited interest will be paid to methodology, so it is unwise to spend a lot of time writing about this. This is one difference between undertaking real-world research and undertaking academic study. For the former it is necessary to spell out, with clarity, what you will be doing and why. For the latter, the theoretical underpinnings of the research design are necessary as part of the academic assessment; this is where the candidate shows conceptual mastery. This is an important distinction; reviewers do get very unhappy and hence possibly hostile wading through fine distinctions between (for example) interpretive and descriptive phenomenology. What they really want to know is what you are going to do with the money you bid for and why. However, the proposal will benefit from a very brief discussion of choice of methodology: specifically, which paradigms you are going to choose for your research (*Key content* → *Chapter 1*). The main examples include positivism, post-positivism and interpretivism.

If you are working within a qualitative framework then the next, more focal, topic would logically be a choice of framework, such as ethnography, phenomenology, grounded theory or action research to guide the project (*Key content* → *Chapter 2*). If using quantitative methods, then the choice of experimental methods (*Key content* → *Chapter 5*), or non-experimental methods (*Key content* → *Chapter 6*) could be introduced. Again, keep it brief, make your choice and justify it!

Writing a proposal Part 4: Research methods

So far the discussion has been quite general (background). But this is the point where it becomes much more focused (focal). Here the proposer spells out exactly what they plan to do. As before, the main split is between quantitative and qualitative methods. Some of the choices for quantitative methods are summarised in Table 9.1.

The proposal is primarily a practical document. Therefore, in addition to outlining the main methods chosen, the practicalities must be included as well. For all these designs a clear timeline must be included. It should be clear who the research team consists of and what their individual roles are. For an experimental design, the choice of independent variable should be linked to the literature review to illustrate the possibility that this new treatment or change to practice might possibly improve outcomes, or is at least is unlikely to worsen them. The dependent variable(s) must similarly be discussed. If you are going to randomise, how would you do this, and if not, why not (this would then become a quasi-experimental design)?

For all experimental designs it is well to consider ethical issues – although typically they are written up in a later section. This means that the research

Table 9.1 Choices for quantitative methods.

Chosen method	Key content →	Main topics to be addressed in proposal
Experimental	Chapter 5	Identification of independent variable(s) and control Randomisation of sample Identification of dependent variable(s)
Quasi-experimental	Chapter 5	Identification of independent variable(s) and control Identification of dependent variable(s) How it departs from a true experimental design and why
Cross-sectional survey	Chapter 6	Development of questionnaire Piloting of questionnaire Include draft questionnaire in appendix
Longitudinal survey	Chapter 6	Development of questionnaire Piloting of questionnaire Time intervals at which questionnaire administered Include draft questionnaire in appendix

team must make a strong case that no one is likely to be harmed in the experiment, and that participants will be kept safe. Ways to do this should be built into the design. The obvious (but not the only) way to do this is by choosing an appropriate control. It is seldom in healthcare that a placebo is acceptable. Instead standard practice, or even better, 'gold standard' practice (i.e. the best current evidence-based practice) should be included as control. Lastly, for survey designs, it is important that the questionnaire to be used is included. This may be difficult to do in a timely fashion, as piloting and revision of versions take time. It might be reasonable to include a draft '90%' finalised version, with a proviso that some further development might be undertaken before the start of the project.

Some of the choices for qualitative methods are summarised in Table 9.2. Central to the quality of the proposal is who will be conducting the research. In qualitative research the researcher is often the research tool. Therefore in order to be an unbiased and objective investigation, it is vital that the researcher be competent in data collection (*Key content* → *Chapter 3*). Thus it is important that the credibility of the researcher is addressed in the

Table 9.2 Choices for qualitative methods.

Chosen method	Key content →	Main topics be addressed in proposal
Interview	Chapter 3	Type of interview to be used Environment in which interviews take place Types of questions/prompts to be used, plus examples Researcher skills How data will be recorded
Focus group interviews	Chapter 3	Size of focus group and strategy for facilitation Environment in which focus group takes place Types of questions/prompts to be used, plus examples Researcher skills How data will be recorded
Observation	Chapter 3	Environment in which observations take place How data will be recorded, including likely categorisations Researcher skills Number of participants to be observed and expected duration of observation
Documentary	Chapter 3	Types of documents to be explored Researcher skills How data will be extracted and recorded

proposal. In qualitative research, Lincoln and Guba's (1985) criterion of credibility may be helpful. This is an exploration of how confident the researcher and reader can be that the research findings are true. Ways to do this could include undertaking study, working with more experienced researchers or undertaking pilot interviews and taking feedback from the interviewees. One final technique is to use a peer debriefing. This involves discussion with other members of the team about the meaning of the findings, again until a consensus is chosen.

A very powerful technique is to include a member check. This is where provisional findings are fed back to participants. They are then encouraged to comment on these. Effectively the researcher is asking: '*This is what I think you said. Is it what you think you said?*' When discrepancies are found, the researcher would then return to the data to clarify and where necessary correct. As for quantitative research, do not neglect the practicalities. It is necessary to identify where the fieldwork will be undertaken and when. Activities such as these should be written into the proposal to illustrate the likelihood of good quality findings being produced.

Again ethical review will be needed before the project starts, so it is important to build good practice into the proposal. For example, if the interviews are to take place in participants' homes, then it is necessary to safeguard the researcher, often through the use of an accepted single worker policy (as used by health visitors, midwives and other professional groups when visiting their clients).

Writing a proposal Part 5: Choice of sampling strategy

Sampling can be included within the methods section, but more often occupies its own section, and generally this is recommended. Within quantitative methods there are a variety of sampling strategies (*Key content* → *Chapter 5*). Traditionally they have been included under the heading of probability sampling, where a formal or scientific attempt to represent a whole population is made. Some of the main choices include:

1. **Random sampling**: each member of the population has the same likelihood of being included in the sample as any other participant.

2. **Stratified random sampling**: a development of random sampling, where within a given grouping (e.g. age group) each member of the group has the same likelihood of being included in the sample as any other member of the group.
3. **Inclusive sampling**: all members within a given group or clinical area are included within the sample – very popular within healthcare research, as it effectively removes sampling bias.

For smaller scale projects, with limited resources, a **purposive**, non-probability sample may be chosen. This is not as strong or rigorous a sampling method, but may be perfectly adequate. In purposive sampling the characteristics to be investigated are identified, and participants who meet these criteria are approached and enrolled in the study.

Within qualitative methods there are similarly a variety of sampling strategies (*Key content → Chapter 3*). In general, these do not attempt to represent a larger population. Rather, in line with the goals of qualitative research, they explore the characteristics of the participants identified in the research question. In general, therefore, they may best be described as broadly fitting within purposive sampling. There are variants, which include:

1. **Quota sampling**: purposive sampling up to a predetermined limit.
2. **Snowball sampling**: this is where a participant is invited to identify someone with a similar profile, who could usefully be included within the project.
3. **Theoretical sampling**: utilised within grounded theory, but useful elsewhere. In this context, a set of data is collected and analysed, and the research team decides whether the research question has been answered in full. If not, then further sampling can be undertaken until the project is complete. This has a major advantage in that, rather than choosing a nominal number of (for example) 12 participants to be involved (there is nothing magical about the number 12), sampling continues until the research question has been fully answered.

When writing the proposal, note that again the reviewers are unlikely to be interested in your theoretical knowledge, so you might be best served by saving that for academic work. A brief statement about the sampling strategy used might be useful, but of greater value is a discussion of who you would include in the research (inclusion criteria) and who you would exclude from the research (exclusion criteria). For example, Pollard (2011, p. 2), used qualitative research to explore the use of a feeding log on breastfeeding. Her **inclusion criteria** were that participants must:

- be first-time mothers
- be between the ages of 18 and 40
- be planning to breast feed
- be able to speak English
- have delivered a healthy infant greater than 37 weeks gestation
- have initiated breastfeeding within 24 hours of delivery

Her sole **exclusion criterion** was mothers who were unable to breastfeed due to a medical condition.

Fortuitously, Pollard (2011) also illustrates an excellent principle; it is a good idea to be sparing in your exclusion criteria. Try to include as many as you can!

Writing a proposal Part 6: Ethics

This section will be split into two parts. The first, ethical considerations, is relatively straightforward. This is where the proposal shows how neither the researcher nor the participant will be put at unnecessary or unjustifiable risk. It is about the application of sensible precautions to the research design. The second part discusses the ethical processes that anyone wishing to conduct research within the NHS must undertake. This is more complex, to the extent that it may be seen as a significant barrier to aspiring researchers. But even so, it is a system which must be dealt with.

Ethical considerations

The application of ethical considerations to qualitative research has already been introduced (*Key content* → *Chapter 4*). This section will present these topics, and others, in an applied way as they might be required in a proposal.

All research contains potential risks for the participants. In some designs, the risks are high-profile and clear. The classic example here would be an experiment, where the participants are given a new treatment. If a new anti-clotting drug were being investigated, it is quite clear that the risks would potentially be huge. If the drug did not work, participants would be at risk of embolic stroke or thromboses, which in a severe case could lead to death. If it worked too well, then the risks, included bleeding disorders such as haemorrhagic stroke and massive blood loss, could also lead to death. To put participants at such risk means that the benefits must potentially be equally large.

Fortunately, most small-scale research projects carry much less risk and so require commensurately less justification. If your project is based around a survey of, for example, how students evaluate their post-registration learning programmes, then it is clear that the risks are much lower. You might even be tempted to say there are no risks (beyond the possibility of an inadvertent paper cut). However, all research projects regardless of design do indeed carry risk, and the proposal needs to show how this risk has been managed. As a minimum, all research projects need to explain how **consent**, **confidentiality** and **safe data management** will be accomplished (Oliver, 2003), plus any specific risks relevant to the project. Currently in the UK, the National Research Ethics Service (NRES) coordinates applications to the NHS and provides guidance for researchers. Much of the content of this and the next section will reflect this guidance. The reader is recommended to explore the NRES (2013) website as it contains much valuable information, but it is quite complex, so some suggestions for navigation are given in Table 9.3.

Consent is a familiar topic for healthcare professionals. All participants within a healthcare research study have the right to give informed consent

Table 9.3 Useful navigation within the NRES (http://www.nres.nhs.uk/) website (2013).

Topic	Navigation	Content
Consent	Homepage → Applications → Guidance → Consent guidance and forms	Consent form template
Participant Information Sheet	Homepage → Applications Guidance → Consent guidance and forms	Information sheet and consent form guidance
Is it research?	Homepage → Applications → Is your project research?	Defining research
Proportionate review	Homepage → Applications → Proportionate review	No Material Ethical Issues Tool

before being involved in any research project. Consent is given in writing and should confirm that:

- The participant understands the research project and specifically what is required of them
- Their participation is voluntary
- They can withdraw at any time
- Any report will not contain information which can be used to identify individuals

For each of these items there should be a box for providing signed initials – note that a tick box is not adequate.

The NRES website provides a downloadable consent form template, plus a very detailed set of guidance. The latter is very important, especially if the research being proposed includes any vulnerable groups such as children, those with mental health problems or learning disability, or prisoners. For all of these groups, and others, special arrangements may be required that are outside of the scope of this book, so the researcher should seek out specialised guidance.

If conducting an anonymised survey, completion of the questionnaire may be taken as implying consent, so no signature may be required – but the researcher should think about how the research is to be conducted. If the researcher gives out the questionnaire and waits for its return, then anonymity is compromised, and this exemption is not reasonable. It applies typically to studies where the questionnaire is sent out by electronic means or by internal or external post and is returned similarly. A detailed Participant Information Sheet will be required to spell out the conditions under which the research will operate.

The Participant (or Patient) Information Sheet

Implicit in the concept of informed consent is the giving of information. This really covers three main aspects: what is required of the participant in the project, what risks are involved, and how these risks are managed. This information is given in the Participant Information Sheet. The main headings commonly used are illustrated in Table 9.4.

Table 9.4 Main headings in the Participant Information Sheet.

Heading	Notes
Invitation to participate	General introduction, giving the title of the study, who is conducting it and which organisation or company they work for
Purpose of the study	*Study-specific*: the main aims presented in layperson's terms. If related to a change in treatment, a brief outline of this would be included
Why have I been invited?	*Study-specific*: this outlines the inclusion criteria, again in layperson's terms
Do I have to take part?	This states clearly that taking part is voluntary, and that no difference will be made to current treatment or conditions of service (for example) if the decision is made *not* to participate
What will happen to me if I take part?	*Study-specific*: a brief discussion of the study and the participant's role
Will I personally benefit from taking part?	Commonly there is no personal benefit from taking part in the study. Ethically this is important and should be stated – otherwise the participant may take part thinking they will receive preferential treatment, which is a form of coercion. Commonly it may be that the findings will help develop care for future patients, and this could reasonably be stated
Possible risks of taking part	In addition to study specific items, safe data management and anonymity can be spelt out here or under their own headings. It is acceptable to say that the study is believed to be of low risk (for survey or interview work for example)

Researcher safety

This is often the poor relative of research proposals, but the researcher should also consider their own safety. This is particularly true if the researcher considers going outside of their place of practice to collect data. If this is the case, then it is advisable to consult the organisation's lone worker policy, which usually contains clauses about signing out and in of the workplace, registering where the data will be collected and how to keep in contact. The organisation may require a risk assessment of the activities, which typically outlines the possible risks to the researcher, how they will be addressed and the potential level of risk. Note that if things do go wrong in the interview, it might be necessary to have the option of a de-brief with a colleague or supervisor to minimise stress and possible emotional damage. This is unlikely perhaps, but be aware of risk if asking sensitive questions or visiting sensitive or vulnerable groups, who may be unpredictable. A very obvious measure which may be employed is to always be accompanied by a colleague.

Finally, it is worth mentioning that when undertaking research, nurses and midwives are, of course, still bound by their code of conduct, specifically the NMC Code (2008), so any actions proposed must be congruent with this too.

Ethical processes: is it research?

This seems an odd question to ask in a book about research. However NRES (and the NHS in general), make a number of distinctions between different categories of inquiry which can be loosely described as 'research'. NRES produce a very helpful document titled 'Defining research' which can be downloaded as shown in Table 9.3. It is advisable to read this thoroughly. This makes the distinction between (i) true research, (ii) service evaluation/development and (iii) clinical audit. The NRES definitions are quite medically skewed, and as so often in the world of ethics, do not provide watertight definitions. There are crossovers between categories – but here is a reasonable interpretation:

- **Research**: Includes all experiments. Any design which involves allocation to a new treatment is included in this category. Qualitative research to explore new themes is also included here.
- **Service evaluation/development**: Includes projects where there is no new allocation to treatment, and where data are collected to identify the current level of service or standard of care. Logically, therefore, if a new aspect of service has *already* been introduced, then qualitative or quantitative exploration of its impact may be included here.
- **Audit**: Collects qualitative or quantitative data to determine whether or not a service reaches a particular standard of care.

This might seem slightly obscure, but for a researcher (as the following section will illustrate) there is a significant benefit in being able to honestly describe their project as 'service development'. By now, the reader will have familiarity with some of the functions of NRES. This organisation also coordinates the NHS Research Ethics Committees (RECs) throughout the UK. There are currently (2013) 100 RECs within the UK. All applications to undertake research within the NHS must be considered by a REC. There are two exceptions to this.

The first of these has already been discussed. If a project can be realistically described as service development, or clinical audit, then it will not have to be taken to a REC. All others will, with the second exception of research involving staff only as participants. Since 2010, the Governance Arrangements for Research Ethics Committees (DH, 2012), identifies (section 2.3.13) that it is the responsibility of employers to safeguard their employees; therefore RECs do not expect to review research which involves staff solely. As this implies, employers also have responsibilities relating to research. In 2005 (later updated in 2010), the Department of Health published its Research Governance Framework (DH, 2010b), which stipulates that all research involving human beings, samples, patient data, NHS staff or facilities must adhere to a set of guidelines. These require scientific rigour, a justified choice of methodology and evidence of the capacity and skills of the researcher (this is why a *curriculum vitae* is often requested of researchers). These should all be integral in a good quality research proposal. Finally, each NHS employer is required to keep a register of all research activity, and authorisation has to be gained from the directors of research within the organisation or trust before the project commences data collection. These activities are commonly carried out within NHS Trusts by the Research and Development (R&D) offices.

This is clearly quite a complex process. Figure 9.2 summarises the main processes involved in applying for ethical approval to commence a research project within the NHS in the UK, as of early 2013.

This is quite a busy diagram, but most of the processes are reasonably straightforward. Firstly, the researcher produces a research proposal, as outlined above. The first stage (1) is informal and will vary according to the institution. In general, it is impossible to undertake a research project without the support of key players within the clinical area. As a minimum, the support of your immediate manager plus an agreement at directorate (or equivalent) level is a good start. It is also worth considering whether the medical manager should be approached. Although the research may not be focused on aspects of medical care, consultant-level medical staff remain key players, and it may be worth getting them onside.

Having done this, it may then be worth reviewing the NRES criteria (2) as to which form of research enquiry requires formal ethical consideration (the 'Is this research' document; see above). If it can be described as service evaluation/development, or audit, then it may be possible to avoid formal ethical

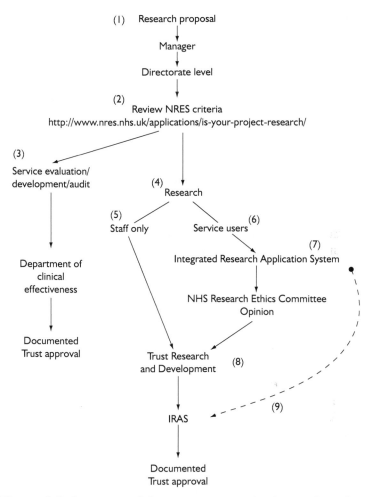

Figure 9.2 Summary of the processes involved in applying for ethical approval.

consideration. If this is the case (3), then within most NHS Trusts there are departments involved in developing practice (for example the 'Department of Clinical Effectiveness' shown in the diagram), and it may be possible to ask them to adopt the project. If this is the case, the project leader should obtain documented approval before proceeding, to show that appropriate governance is in place for their own protection.

If the project is judged to be true research, then a decision is made as to whether the participants are staff only, or involve patients or clients or carers (4). If staff only are involved (5), then the NHS Trust R&D office can be approached. The office will advise the researcher as to the local processes that are required to obtain permission to proceed. This may involve completing the Integrated Research Application System (IRAS) form (see the following section).

If service users are participants in the research (6), then the researcher must complete the IRAS form (7). This is administered by NRES and is an electronic form. It must be completed online, as various parts of the form are activated or de-activated according to the research design. It is possible to set up an IRAS account on line for free (https://www.myresearchproject. org.uk/Signin.aspx), but it is commonly agreed that for inexperienced (and indeed experienced) researchers the IRAS form is technically very difficult and time-consuming. First-time users are strongly advised to have an experienced researcher to help with this. Trust R&D offices can also be extremely helpful with IRAS (and indeed other aspects of the ethical process), so it is worth spending some time forming positive relations with the people who work in the office.

Once the IRAS form has been completed, NRES will book the proposal into a suitable REC, usually within the same county (8). The researcher will be invited to attend the REC meeting. If so, this is very worthwhile, and although usually quite stressful, can save a lot of correspondence and potential delay. There is an exception to this, called Proportionate Review. Details of this can be accessed using the directions given in Table 9.3. A proposal is considered within Proportionate Review when it is agreed that there are 'no material ethical issues' involved. Typically this includes research which uses non-experimental designs, including surveys and interviews of non-sensitive topics, to groups who are not vulnerable. Proportionate review is conducted by a subgroup of the REC, and can be very rapid indeed. Although attendance is not required, it is expected that the researcher will be able to be contacted by telephone for when the review is scheduled. In most cases, the REC will have some questions and may ask for further clarification or changes to the proposal. It is also possible that after amendment it may be necessary to resubmit the proposal, which can be time-consuming. It is best to budget for at least three months and possibly up to six months for the ethics process; on rare occasions it may take up to a year.

Once a favourable review has been given, the researcher can formally approach the Trust R&D office (8). Note that a favourable opinion means that the research is ethically sound. It does not imply that the researcher has any right to actually start the research. This remains at the discretion of the NHS Trust. Given that at any stage in this process permission may be refused, the wise researcher will make early positive contacts with their Trust R&D Office (9). Experience has taught that these people are the gatekeepers of the NHS research world, are often very helpful, and are well worth getting to know!

Running your small-scale research project – a series of logical steps

Once you have decided to undertake a small-scale research project, prepared your proposal, submitted your bid for research funding and have the funding secured, you are committed to undertaking the highest quality research possible, within your funding envelope and your time frame. The steps below are designed to ensure you are successful in achieving your research outcomes, and to minimise the chances of mishaps in the research process. However, should these occur (and they do, as all experienced researchers will tell you) simply revert to this guide and repeat/revisit the step immediately prior to the point where your project experienced a difficulty.

1. Identify your team

Step 1 is vital, hence its position at the start of this guide. Identification of research team members can present a number of challenges, which, if not thought through at the beginning of the process, can lead to difficulties later on. Broadly speaking, these challenges are related to personal issues (we return to this later) for example multiple locations, distance from the main site of the research study, and professional disciplines which might come into conflict. Communication is absolutely key to ensuring you have the right people on the team. In practical terms you will need to consider where your research is located in relation to your team members and the funding you have acquired for travel, subsistence and general expenses. To return to an earlier point, it is imperative that your research project has been properly costed, as it is unlikely that your funders will increase funding once the project has been accepted.

The expectation is that you have thought this through and requested the funds you will need to cover the cost of project delivery, including expenses for the research team.

On a personal note, clearly research team members need to engage with and be able to work with each other. Personality clashes within teams are not helpful in achieving the aims of the research project and it is worth thinking about working relationships at the outset. Researchers do quite often fall out with each other, especially as deadlines loom. Again, communication is key in decisions regarding who is responsible for what, and this is addressed in detail below.

One note of caution here is always to address the issue of authorship or outputs and acknowledgement of effort at an early stage in the project, as these are important considerations given the significance of outputs and their impact on research careers. There are conventions relating to authorship, which are helpful within a given discipline. However, what is perhaps more important is to gain the agreement of all team members regarding how you wish to approach authorship. For example, it is usual for all participating research team members to be included in any publication/output, with the Principal Investigator's (PI) name appearing first. However, as a research team you may agree for another team member to 'lead' on a particular publication, with their name subsequently appearing first on the paper, i.e. represented as lead author. In this example the PI may appear as last-named author on the paper to indicate they are the PI, with other contributors appearing in alphabetical order. For example in the paper by Dyson, S. E., Atkin, K., Culley, L., Demaine, J. and Dyson, S. M. (2012) entitled 'School ethos and variation in health experience of young people with sickle cell disorder at school', Dyson, S. E., a team member, took the lead in writing the paper and is duly acknowledged as first author, with contributing research team members appearing in alphabetical order, and Dyson, S. M., the PI, appearing last. Whatever the convention followed (and it may be quite different within a given discipline), what is important is a consensus on the protocol to be followed.

2. Decide who is responsible for what

Step 2 of this practical guide to small project management is also crucial in that each team member will need to know what role you expect them to fulfil within the overall research team. For example, a team member may be part of the project due to their subject expertise and may have agreed to participate in the research project on this basis. While this seems common sense, a project can come unstuck if team members are unaware of the remit of other colleagues, and expectations are at odds with what is subsequently delivered. Your role here as project lead, or PI, is to determine, with consensus, the roles and responsibilities of each research team member and to formally communicate this to the team.

3. How often will you meet?

Research team members will need to know the location of all the meetings they are expected to attend and/or the location of data collection if they are involved in this. Frequency, dates and times of meetings need to be set well in advance in order to maximise attendance of team members and to fit in with busy diaries and workloads. It is imperative that you, as project lead, ensure that the research team can fulfil their roles in order that research objectives are achieved. You are ultimately responsible to your funders, who will require interim and final reports, including an account and/or audit of how monies have been spent. Most research funders draw on public money and researchers and funders have a duty to account fully for how this money is spent.

4. Project governance

The decision about whether to have a steering group or project group or both is the responsibility of the PI to determine. The PI is named as such on the bid, with other members of the research team identified as co-applicants. The PI is responsible for overseeing the running of the research project and ensuring its overall success, part of which is reporting regularly to the funding body. The running of the research project and how this is to be organised depends on the size of the project, the number of researchers engaged on the project and whether or not external expertise is required, i.e. individuals who will not be part of the day-to-day research but who have expertise in the subject or discipline, or represent a body of people (for example service users, carers and/or practice).

A steering group can serve an essential function in project governance. They afford a formal meeting where management decisions concerning the research are made and/or reported on and should be officially recorded. Project governance is a critical element of any research project, irrespective of the size, extent and scope of the research, because accountability and responsibility will need to be officially recognised and recorded. The steering group is the group that determines the structure of the project or research plan including the time frame and agreed deliverables (outputs). It details who within the research team is responsible for each part of the project (for example literature review, data collection, transcription, analysis). The steering group will need to identify a single person or point of accountability.

Accountability for the success of the project depends on strong and clear leadership. Having a single person identified as accountable for project delivery will go a long way to ensuring success of the project in almost all situations. However, should issues arise that have an effect on the overall success or delivery of the aims and objectives of the research, then the named and recognised accountable person will need to make and take sound decisions. While a collective and collaborative approach to decision-making is essential for team cohesion, nevertheless someone will need to take overall responsibility for leading the research team.

Finally, the steering group will need to determine who owns the research. What we mean here is an agreement and understanding of an organisation's role and expectation regarding the research. For example, research projects can be collaborations between organisations, often but not exclusively involving universities and the NHS and the private and/or voluntary sectors. These organisations are often referred to as the 'stakeholders' in the project. The intended recipients of the research (for example service users or practice colleagues) may also be deemed to be stakeholders. However many partners or collaborators are included in the research, all will have expectations regarding the outcomes and impact of the project. One area where this is extremely important is that of intellectual property and who owns this. The steering group will need to address the question of ownership at an early stage of the project and may need to consult with experts (for example an organisation's legal team or R&D department) in order to ensure that the correct procedures have been considered and the issue of ownership of the research has been resolved to the satisfaction of all parties.

5. Terms of reference

Terms of reference are required to describe the purpose and structure of the research project and are agreed by the steering group members who have agreed to work together to achieve the aims and objectives of the research. The terms of reference can be broadly described as the research project charter. Detailed terms of reference will ensure that the vision for the research is achieved. The list below sets out the essential elements contained within the terms of reference of a research project steering group:

- Vision, objectives, scope and deliverables (i.e. what has to be achieved)
- Stakeholders, roles and responsibilities (i.e. who will take part in it)
- Resources, financial and quality plans (i.e. how it will be achieved)
- Work breakdown structure and schedule (i.e. when it will be achieved)

6. Project plan and project team

Step 6 essentially concerns the project itself and commences once the other steps have been completed. The research project now depends on the project team fulfilling their roles and responsibilities as determined by the research steering group. Project team members may or may not be steering group members or may be co-opted onto the steering group as and when required, for example to report on project progress, or to request support when a decision is required to revise the project in light of events. The role of the project team is to undertake the elements of the research process within a given area of responsibility in the specified time frame, which will have been identified, agreed and recorded in a project plan. A simple version of a project plan is shown in Table 9.5. However, you may want to develop your own, which as a

Table 9.5 A simple project plan.

Activity	Responsibility	Due by	Progress	Notes	Completed
Literature review	Researcher 1	1 September	First draft available	First draft of literature review presented to steering group on...	
Research sample frame	Researcher 2	31 September	Sampling strategies under consideration	Sampling strategy agreed by steering group on...	
Data collection	Researcher 2	To commence 1 October			

minimum should identify the activity, the person responsible for the activity, and when the activity will be completed.

7. Achieving objectives and reporting to funders

The aim of all projects is to achieve the research objectives and to make a difference in some way. This might be a relatively small change in practice, or a different way of thinking about a thorny issue, or it might be a significant change to a way of thinking about a major issue required or a significant policy change, for example a recently completed research project looked at how children with sickle cell disease are supported at school (Dyson *et al.*, 2010). This project was funded by the Economic and Social Research Council (ESRC), the UK's largest organisation for funding research on economic and social issues. The project team developed a guide to school policy which advised schools on how to support children with sickle cell disease based on the findings of the research team. The ESRC required a comprehensive and full report detailing the project outcomes, deliverables and impact. For more information on this see Economic and Social Research Council (2011). All funding bodies will require some form of report, although this may be in different formats, which you will need to be familiar with, and may include some form of progress reporting or interim report. It is the responsibility of the PI, supported by the project team and overseen by the steering group, to ensure reporting requirements are adhered to.

8. Finishing and/or winding up the project

It is important to have a well-considered strategy for dissemination of your research findings. In many ways this signals the conclusion of the research project and/or the entering of the final stage, although you may have engaged in interim dissemination throughout the project if the research team believe there are important early findings or insights which need to be shared and placed in the public domain before the project officially concludes. A number of considerations are important when thinking about a dissemination plan or strategy: for example, how will your findings be disseminated and through which medium? Some possibilities include:

- Professional conferences
- Media coverage
- Press release
- Research summary document
- Flyers, posters, brochures, and research briefing papers
- Policy briefs
- Study newsletters
- Community agency publications and websites and list servers
- Local events, seminars, conferences, community meetings
- Letters of thanks to study participants
- Publications in subject-specific journals or practice-focused journals

Arguably the first priority in any dissemination plan is returning the results to the study participants. This is followed by dissemination to any stakeholder group. To be effective it is important that any dissemination plan has been formulated early and has the full agreement of the steering group members and the project team. When thinking through the dissemination strategy a good place to start is to define the goal of your particular projects, i.e. what is the goal and the objective of your strategy and what impact do you hope to have? Once you have considered this you can identify from the (non-exhaustive) list above the medium for dissemination. You will need to consider your audience, i.e. who is affected by your research and who will be interested to know of your findings. Finally, you will want to consider when to execute your dissemination plan, for example at which points during the study (if you decide to disseminate early), and afterwards, and who will be responsible for each dissemination activity.

Very small projects

As you can see, conducting a funded research project can be complex and quite daunting. There are, fortunately, two remedies for this. Firstly, you may wish to start small. Quite often bodies such as NHS Trusts or universities may have small pots of money available within a service, from donations from satisfied customers, from local charities or from legacies. If this is the case, a modest sum (for example £1,000) could allow an individual to undertake a small project, write it up, and publish the results. This may not produce earth-shattering research, but it may be enough to move practice within your area forward by an increment, and it will give you valuable experience of running a (very) small-scale project. The other option is to attach yourself to an existing project within your clinical area. You may be aware of research groups or research active staff within your clinical area. Rather than initially running the project, you may wish to become part of an already viable team. Most research teams will welcome people who are interested, but before agreeing to a significant investment of your time, be aware of the issues surrounding authorship, as outlined above.

In conclusion, this chapter has provided you with a practical guide to submitting a research bid, writing your research proposal, managing your research project and sharing, through a clear approach to dissemination, your important research findings. It remains only for us to encourage you to 'have a go', which is the spirit in which this chapter was written. Remember, even though a high proportion of research bids are not funded, those most definitely not funded are those which are never submitted.

References

Andrews-Fike, C. (1999) A review of postpartum depression. *Journal of Clinical Psychiatry*, **1**(1), 9–14.

Anthony, D. (1996) A review of statistical methods in the *Journal of Advanced Nursing*. *Journal of Advanced Nursing*, **24**(5), 1089–94.

Anthony, D. (1999) *Understanding Advanced Statistics*. Churchill Livingstone, London.

Argyrous, G. (2005) *Statistics for Research With a Guide to SPSS*, 2nd edn. Sage, Thousand Oaks, CA.

Ashing-Giwa, K.T., Padilla, G., Tejero, J., Kraemer, J., Wright, K., Coscarelli, A., Clayton, S., Williams, I., Hills, D. (2002) Understanding the breast cancer experience of women: a qualitative study of African American, Asian American, Latina and Caucasian cancer survivors. *Psycho-oncology*, **13**(6), 408–28.

Bannigan, K. and Watson, R. (2009) Reliability and validity in a nutshell. *Journal of Clinical Nursing*, **18**, 3237–43.

Barker, S. (2010) The Midwife's Coracle: a phenomenological study of midwives' experiences of emotionally supporting motherhood. *PhD thesis*. http://eprints. bournemouth.ac.uk/13820/ (accessed 5 May 2013).

Benner, P. (1984) From novice to expert: excellence and power in clinical nursing practice. *The American Journal of Nursing*, **84**(12), 1480.

Bjelland, I., Dahl, A., Haug, T., Neckelmann, D. (2002) The validity of the Hospital Anxiety and Depression Scale. An updated literature review. *Journal of Psychosomatic Research,* **52**(2): 69–77.

Bournemouth University (2013) *Research Blog*. Available from: http://blogs. bournemouth.ac.uk/research/tag/grant-writing/ (accessed 2 May 2013).

Bowling, A. (2009) *Research Methods in Health: Investigating Health and Health Services*, 3rd edn. Open University Press, Buckingham.

Bowling, A. and Ibrahim, S. (2005) *Handbook of Health Research Methods*. Open University Press, Maidenhead.

Bryar, R. (1999) An examination of case study research. *Nurse Researcher*, **7**(2), 61–78.

Buchbinder, R. Kallmes, D. and Glasziou, P. (2010) Vertebroplasty versus conservative treatment for vertebral fractures (2007). *Lancet*, **376**(9746), 1085–92; **376** (9758), 2070-2.

Campbell, K. (2006) *Myeloproliferative Disorders*. Leukaemia Research, London.

Carr, W. and Kemmis, S. (1986) *Becoming Critical. Education, Knowledge and Action Research*. Falmer, Lewes.

Clarke, M., Hopewell, S., Juszczak, E., Eisinga, A. and Kjeldstrøm, M. (2006) Compression stockings for preventing deep vein thrombosis in airline passengers. *Cochrane Database of Systematic Reviews*, Issue 2. Art. No.: CD004002. DOI: 10.1002/14651858.CD004002.pub2.

Cleave, C. (2009) *The Other Hand*. Sceptre, London.

Cohen, J. (1988) *Statistical Power Analysis for the Behavioral Sciences*, 2nd edn. Erlbaum Associates, London.

Cott, N. F. (1987) *The Grounding of Modern Feminism*. Yale University Press, New Haven.

Cox, J. Holden, J. and Sagovsky, R. (1987) Detection of postnatal depression: development of the 10-item Edinburgh Postnatal Depression Scale. *British Journal of Psychiatry*, **150**, 782–6.

Crozier, K. (2009) *Royal College of Midwives. Innovation and Research in Midwifery*. Available from: http://www.rcm.org.uk/midwives/in-depth-papers/innovation-and-research-in-midwifery/ (accessed 30 April 2013).

Denscombe, M. (2007) *The Good Research Guide: for Small-scale Social Research Projects*, 3rd edn. Open University Press, Maidenhead.

Denzin, N. and Lincoln, Y. (2000) *Handbook of Qualitative Research*, 2nd edn. Sage, Thousand Oaks, CA.

Department of Health (2000) *The NHS Plan*. Crown Copyright. London.

Department of Health (2010a) *Liberating the NHS: Developing the Healthcare Workforce*. Available from: https://www.gov.uk/government/uploads/system/uploads/attachment_data/file/153233/dh_129702pdf.pdf (accessed 4 May 2013).

Department of Health (2010b) *Research Governance Framework for Health and Social Care*, 2nd edn. Available from: http://www.dh.gov.uk/en/Publication-sandstatistics/Publications/PublicationsPolicyAndGuidance/DH_4108962 (accessed 19 April 2013).

Department of Health (2012) *Governance Arrangements for Research Ethics Committees*. Available from: https://www.gov.uk/government/uploads/system/uploads/attachment_data/file/135218/dh_133993.pdf.pdf (accessed 19 April 2013).

DeVon, H., Block, M., Moyle Wright, P., Ernst, D., Hayden, S., Lazarra, D., Savoy, S. and Kostas Polston, E. (2007) A psychometric toolbox for testing validity and reliability. *Journal of Nursing Scholarship*, **39**(2), 155–64.

Dick, B. (2005) *Grounded Theory: A Thumbnail Sketch*. Resource papers in action research. http://www.scu.edu.au/schools/gcm/ar/arp/grounded/.

Doll, R. Peto, R. and Sutherland, I. (2004) Mortality in relation to smoking: 50 years' observation on male British doctors. *British Medical Journal,* **328**(7455), 1519.

Dyson, S. E. (2005) Global boarders: Leaving Zimbabwe – factors influencing undergraduate student's decision to study nursing in the UK. In: *Health Economics Management and Policy* (eds. J. N. Yfantopoulos and G. T. Papanikos), pp. 135–72. Athens Institute for Education and Research, Athens.

Dyson, S. and Brown, B. (2006). *Social Theory and Applied Health Research.* Open University Press, Berkshire.

Dyson, S., Culley, L., Gill, C., Hubbard, S., Kennefick, A., Morris, P., Sutton, F., Squire, P. (2006) Ethnicity questions and antenatal screening for sickle cell/ thalassaemia [EQUANS] in England: a randomized controlled trial of two questionnaires. *Ethnicity and Health,* **11**(2), 169–89.

Dyson, S., Culley, L., Norrie, P. and Genders, N. (2008) An exploration of the experiences of South Asian students on pre-registration nursing. *Journal of Research in Nursing,* **13**(2), 163–76.

Dyson, S. M., Abuateya, H., Atkin, K., Culley, L. A., Dyson, S. E. and Rowley, D. T. (2010) Reported school experiences of young people living with sickle cell disorder in England. *British Educational Research Journal,* **36**(1), 125–42.

Dyson, S. E., Atkin, K., Culley, L., Demaine, J. and Dyson, S. M. (2012) School ethos and variation in health experience of young people with sickle cell disorder at school. *Diversity and Equality in Health and Care,* **9**(1), 33–44.

Economic and Social Research Council (2011) *Education for Minority Ethnic Pupils: Young People with Sickle Cell Disease.* Available from: http://www. esrc.ac.uk/my-esrc/grants/RES-000-23-1486/read (accessed 4 April 2013).

Elenbaas, R., McNabney, W. and Robinson, W. (1984) Evaluation of prophylactic oxacillin in dog bite wounds. *Annals of Emergency Medicine,* **13**(3), 155–7.

Field, A. (2009) *Discovering Statistics Using SPSS,* 3rd edn. Sage, Thousand Oaks, CA.

Fink, A. (1995) *How to Ask Survey Questions.* Sage, Thousand Oaks, CA.

Finlay, L. (2008) A dance between the reduction and reflexivity: explicating the 'phenomenological psychological attitude'. *Journal of Phenomenological Psychology,* **39**, 1–32.

Frei, H., Everts, R., Von Ammon, K., Kaufmann, F., Walther, D., Schmitz, S. F., Collenberg, M., Steinlin, M., Lim, C. and Thurneysen, A. (2007) Randomised controlled trials of homeopathy in hyperactive children: treatment procedure leads to an unconventional study design. Experience with open-label homeopathic treatment preceding the Swiss ADHD placebo controlled, randomised, double-blind, cross-over trial. *Homeopathy,* **96**(1), 35–41.

Fowler, J. and Norrie, P. (2009) Development of an attrition risk prediction. *British Journal of Nursing,* **18**(19), 1194–200.

Geertz, C. (1973) *The Interpretation of Cultures: Selected Essays.* Basic Books, New York.

Gillham, B. (2000a) *Developing a Questionnaire.* Continuum, New York.

Gillham, B. (2000b) *Case Study Research Methods.* Continuum, London.

Glaser, B. (1978) *Theoretical Sensitivity: Advances in the Methodology of Grounded Theory.* Sociology Press, California.

Glaser, B. G. and Strauss, A. L. (1967) *The Discovery of Grounded Theory: Strategies for Qualitative Research.* Aldine, Chicago.

Glasziou, P., Del Mar, C. and Salisbury, J. (2003) *Evidence Based Medicine Workbook.* BMJ Books, London.

Grbich, C. (2004) *New Approaches in Social Research.* Sage, London.

Greasley, P. (2008) *Quantitative Data Analysis Using SPSS: an Introduction for Health and Social Science.* Open University Press, New York.

Grey, M. (2009) *Evidence Based Healthcare and Public Health*, 3rd edn. Churchill Livingstone, Edinburgh.

Guyatt, G. H., Sackett, D. L., Sinclair, J. C., Hayward, R., Cook, D. J. and Cook, R. J. (1995) Users' guides to the medical literature; a method for grading health care recommendations. *Journal of the American Medical Association*, **274**, 1800–4.

Hammersley, M. (1990) *Classroom Ethnography: Empirical and Methodological Essays.* Open University Press, Milton Keynes.

Harrison, C. N., Campbell, P. J., Buck, G., Wheatley, K., East, C. L., Bareford, D., Wilkins, B. S., van der Walt, J. D., Reilly, J. T., Grigg, A. P., Revell, P., Woodcock, B. E. and Green, A. R. (2005) Hydroxyurea compared with anagrelide in high-risk essential thrombocythaemia. *New England Journal of Medicine*, **353**(1), 33–45.

Hay, I. (2005) *Qualitative Research Methods in Human Geography*, 2nd edn. Oxford University Press, Oxford.

Hersey, J. C., Khavjou, O., Strange, L. B., Atkinson, R. L., Blair, S. N., Campbell, S., Hobbs, C. L., Kelly, B., Fitzgerald, T. M., Kish-Doto, J., Koch, M. A., Munoz, B., Peele, E., Stockdale, J., Hersey, J., Kelly, B., Roussel, A., LaShawn, C., Horne, J., Williams-Piehota, P., Kuester, S. and Farris, R. (2012) The value of partnerships in state obesity prevention and control programs. *Health Promotion Practice*, **13**(2), 222–9.

Holloway, I. (1997) *Basic Concepts for Qualitative Research.* Blackwell Science, Oxford.

Holloway, I. and Walker, J. (2000) *Getting a PhD in Health and Social Care.* Blackwell Science, Oxford.

Hughes, M. A., Deery, R. and Lovatt, A. (2002) A critical ethnographic approach to facilitating cultural shift in midwifery. *Midwifery*, **18**(1), 43–52.

Husserl, E. (1970) *Logical Investigations* (transl. D. Carr). Humanities Press, New York.

Joanna Briggs Institute (2012a) *Joanna Briggs Institute (Homepage)*. Available from: http://www.joannabriggs.edu.au/ (accessed 18 February 2013).

Joanna Briggs Institute (2012b) *Levels of Evidence FAME*. Available from: http://www.joannabriggs.edu.au/Levels%20of%20Evidence%20%20FAME (accessed 18 February 2013).

Kallmes, D., Comstock, B., Heagerty, P., Turner, J., Wilson, D., Diamond, T., Edwards, R., Gray, L., Stout, L., Owen, S., Hollingworth, W., Ghdoke, B., Annesley-Williams, D., Ralston, S. and Jarvik, J. (2009) A randomized controlled trial of vertebroplasty for osteoporotic compression fractures. *New England Journal of Medicine*, **361**, 569–79.

Keating, A. and Fleming, V. E. (2009) Midwives' experiences of facilitating normal birth in an obstetric-led unit: a feminist perspective. *Midwifery*, **25**(5), 518–27.

Kennedy, H. P., Erickson-Owens, D. and Davis, J. A. (2006) Voices of diversity in midwifery: a qualitative research study. *Journal of Women's Health*, **51**(2), 85–90.

Key, J. (1997) *Research Design in Occupational Education: Qualitative Research* (Module 14). Available at http://www.okstate.edu/ag/agedcm4h/academic/aged5980a/5980/newpage21.htm; accessed 25 April 2010.

Kirkham, M. and Stapleton, H. (2000) Midwives' support needs as childbirth changes. *Journal of Advanced Nursing*, **32**(2), 465–72.

Kitto, S., Chesters, J. and Grbich, C. (2008) Quality in qualitative research. *Medical Journal of Australia*, **188**(4), 243–6.

Knowles, M. S. (1998) *The Adult Learner: a Neglected Species*, 5th edn. Gulf, Houston.

Kunz, R., Vist, G. and Oxman, A. (2007) Randomisation to protect against selection bias in healthcare trials. *Cochrane Database of Systematic Reviews 2007*, Issue 2. Article No.: MR000012.

Lester, S. (1999) *An Introduction to Phenomenological Research*. Stan Lester Developments, Taunton.

Lewins, A., Taylor, C. and Gibbs, G. R. (2005) *What is Qualitative Data Analysis (QDA)?* Available at: http://onlineqda.hud.ac.uk/Intro_QDA/what_is_qda. php; Accessed 25 April 2010.

Lincoln, Y. and Guba, E. (1985) *Naturalistic Enquiry*. Sage, Thousand Oaks.

McNiff, J. and Whitehead, J. (2006) *All You Need to Know About Action Research*. Sage, Thousand Oaks, CA.

McSherry, R., Simmons, M. and Abbott, P. (2002) *Evidence Informed Nursing: A Guide*. Routledge, London.

Medeiros, I. M. and Saconato, H. (2001) Antibiotic prophylaxis for mammalian bites. *Cochrane Database of Systematic Reviews*, Issue 2. Art. No.: CD001738. DOI: 10.1002/14651858.CD001738.

Merleau-Ponty, M. (1962) *Phenomenology of Perception* (transl. C. Smith). Routledge & Kegan Paul, London. (Original work published 1945.)

Miles, B. and Huberman, M. (1994) *Qualitative Data Analysis: An Expanded Sourcebook*, 2nd edn. Sage, Thousand Oaks, CA.

Morgan, D. L. (1997) *Focus Groups as Qualitative Research*. Sage, London.

Morton-Cooper, A. (2000) *Action Research in Health Care*. Blackwell Science, Oxford.

Mulrow, C. D., Cook, C. (1998) *Systematic Reviews: Synthesis of Best Evidence for Health Care Decisions*. American College of Physicians, Philadelphia.

Munro, B. H. (2005) *Statistical Methods for Health Care Research*. 5th edn. Lippincott Williams & Wilkins, London.

Murray, S. and Graham, L. (1995) Practice-based health needs assessment: use of four methods in a small neighbourhood. *British Medical Journal*, **308**, 1443–8.

National Research Ethics Service (2013) *Homepage*. Available from: http://www.nres.nhs.uk/ (accessed 12 March 2013).

NICE (2007) *Antenatal and Post Natal Mental Health* (CG45). Available from: http://publications.nice.org.uk/antenatal-and-postnatal-mental-health-cg45/introduction (accessed 12 February 2013).

NICE (2008) *Guide to the Methods of Technology Appraisal*. Available from: (http://www.nice.org.uk/media/B52/A7/TAMethodsGuideUpdatedJune2008.pdf (accessed 11 February 2013).

Norrie, P. (1997) Time utilisation of nurses in intensive care. *Nursing in Critical Care*, **2**(3), 121–5.

Norrie, P. (2003) What do critical care nurses want from clinical information systems? *Information Technology in Nursing*, **15**(4), 10–15.

Norrie, P. (2004) Expanding the case study, the narrative thread. *NT Research*, **9**(1), 30–7.

Norrie, P. and Dalby, D. (2007) How adult are our students? A cross sectional exploration of the learning characteristics of nursing students in a United Kingdom university. *Journal of Research in Nursing*, **12**(4), 319–29.

Norrie, P. and Anthony, D. (2004) Are clinical information systems acceptable to critical care nurses? Some findings and a reliable and valid tool for further research peer reviewed research paper. *Information Technology in Nursing*, **16**(1), 12–18.

Nursing and Midwifery Council (2008) *The Code: Standards of Conduct, Performance and Ethics for Nurses and Midwives*. Available from: http://www.nmc-uk.org/Publications/Standards/The-code/Introduction/ (accessed 13 April 2013).

O'Cathain, A., Murphy, E. and Nicholl, J. (2008) The quality of mixed methods studies in health services research. *Journal of Health Services Research & Policy*, **13**(2), 92–8.

Oliver, P (2003) *The Student's Guide to Research Ethics.* Open University Press, Maidenhead.

Oppenheim, A. N. (1992) *Questionnaire Design, Interviewing and Attitude Measurement.* Pinter, London.

Pallant, J. (2010) *SPSS Survival Manual: a Step by Step Guide to Data Analysis Using SPSS,* 4th edn. Open University Press, Maidenhead.

Parahoo, K. (2006) *Nursing Research, Principles, Processes and Issues,* 2nd edn. Palgrave Macmillan, Basingstoke.

Peden, V. and Saddington, C. (2001) Using the Oucher Scale. *Paediatric Nursing,* **13**(3), 24–6.

Phillips, E. and Pugh, D. (2005) *How to get a PhD: a Handbook for Students and Their Supervisors,* 4th edn. Open University Press Buckingham.

Polit, D. F. and Beck, C. T. (2008) *Nursing Research: Generating and Assessing Evidence for Nursing Practice,* 8th edn. Lippincott, Williams & Wilkins, London.

Polkinghorne, D. (1988) *Narrative Knowing and the Human Sciences.* University of New York Press, New York.

Pollard, D. (2011) Impact of a feeding log on breastfeeding duration and exclusivity. *Maternal and Child Health Journal,* **15**(3), 395–400.

Pope, C. and Mays, N. (2000) *Qualitative Research in Health Care,* 2nd edn. BMJ Books, London.

Quality Metric (2013) *The SF Community.* Available from: http://www.sf-36.org (accessed 6 May 2013).

Riessman, C. (1993) *Narrative Analysis.* Qualitative Research Methods Volume 30. Sage, London.

Rosenbaum, M. (2006) Was drug trial payment too high? Available from http://www.bbc.co.uk/blogs/opensecrets/2006/11/tgn1412.html (accessed 23 December 2009).

Royal College of Nursing (2003) *Strategic Plan.* Available from: http://www.rcn.org.uk/__data/assets/pdf_file/0005/78566/001987.pdf (accessed 4 May 2013).

Ryan, K., Brown, S., Wilkins, C., Taylor, A., Arnold, R., Angell, C. and van Teijlingen, E. (2011) Which hat am I wearing today? Practising midwives doing research. *Evidence Based Midwifery,* **9**(1), 4–8.

Sackett, D. L., Rosenberg, W. M., Gray, J. A., Haynes, R. B., Richardson, W. S. (1996) Evidence based medicine: what it is and what it isn't. *British Medical Journal,* **312**(7023), 71–2.

Sapsford, R. (2007) *Survey Research,* 2nd edn. Sage, London.

Sarantakos, S. (2005) *Social Research,* 3rd edn. Palgrave MacMillan, Basingstoke.

Seidal, J. V. (1998) *Qualitative Data Analysis.* Available from http://www.scribd.com/doc/7129360/Seidel-1998-Qualitative-Data-Analysis/ (accessed 25 April 2010).

Shields, L. and Twycross, A. (2008) Sampling in quantitative research. *Paediatric Nursing*, **20**(5), 37.

Sibbald, B. (1998) Understanding controlled trials: Crossover trials. *British Medical Journal*, **316**, 1719.

Sim, J. and Sharp, K. (1998) A critical appraisal of the role of triangulation in nursing research. *International Journal of Nursing Studies*, **35**(1), 23–31.

Sim, J. and Wright, C. (2000) *Research in Health Care. Concepts, Designs and Methods*. Stanley Thornes, Cheltenham.

Sinclair, M. (2011) Research ethics: issues for midwives. *Evidence Based Midwifery*, **9**(1), 3.

Smith, P., James, T., Lorentzon, M. and Pope, R. (2004) *Shaping the Facts: Evidence Based Nursing and Health Care*. Elsevier, Edinburgh.

Talluri, S. K. (2005) Number needed to treat (or harm). *World Journal of Surgery*, **29**(5), 576–81.

Teddlie, C. and Tashakkori, A. (2009) *Foundations of Mixed Methods Research: Integrating Quantitative and Qualitative Approaches in the Social and Behavioural Sciences*. Sage, Thousand Oaks, CA.

Thomas, M., McKinley, R., Mellor, S., Watkin, G., Holloway, E., Scullion, J., Shaw, D., Wardlaw, A., Price, D. and Pavord, I. (2009) Breathing exercises for asthma: a randomised controlled trial. *Thorax*, **64**, 55–61.

Toscano, S.E. (2007) A grounded theory of female adolescents' dating experiences and factors influencing safety: the dynamics of the Circle. *BMC Nursing*, **6**, 7.

Wadsworth, Y. (1998) *What is Action Research?* Action Research International. Available from http://www.scu.edu.au/schools/gcm/ar/ari/p-ywadsworth98.html (accessed 25 April 2010).

Wallis, M. and Tyson, S. (2003) Improving the nursing management of patients in a hematology/oncology day unit: an action research project. *Cancer Nursing*, **26**(1), 75–83.

Walsh, D. and Downe, S. (2005) Meta-synthesis method for qualitative research: a literature review. *Journal of Advanced Nursing*, **50**(2), 204–11.

Yin, R. (2009) *Case Study Research: Design and Methods*, 4th edn. Sage, Thousand Oaks, CA.

Zigmond, A. and Snaith, R. (1983) The Hospital Anxiety and Depression Scale. *Acta Psychiatrica Scandinavica*, **67**, 361–70.

Index